Injury Recognition and Prevention

Injury Recognition and Prevention

Lower and Upper Extremity

Genevieve Ludwig and Megan Streveler

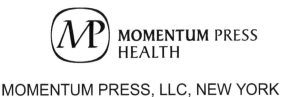

MOMENTUM PRESS HEALTH

MOMENTUM PRESS, LLC, NEW YORK

Injury Recognition and Prevention: Lower and Upper Extremity

Copyright © Momentum Press, LLC, 2016.

First published in 2016 by
Momentum Press, LLC
222 East 46th Street, New York, NY 10017
www.momentumpress.net

ISBN-13: 978-1-94474-939-2 (paperback)
ISBN-13: 978-1-94474-940-8 (e-book)

Momentum Press Health, Wellness, and Exercise Science Collection

Cover and interior design by Exeter Premedia Services Private Ltd., Chennai, India

First edition: 2016

10 9 8 7 6 5 4 3 2 1

Printed in the United States of America.

Abstract

Injury Recognition and Prevention: Lower and Upper Extremity covers the most common musculoskeletal injuries of the arms, legs, and spine. The text is designed to be a reference tool for students and professionals who work with athletes or a physically active population. Each chapter covers a specific anatomical joint area and includes a brief review of musculoskeletal anatomy, common injury etiology, signs and symptoms for easy recognition, and the most commonly prescribed treatment or rehabilitation plan. Also discussed are preventative measures to avoid sustaining these common injuries. Coaches, students in allied health professions, physical education teachers, parents, and athletes will benefit from reading this text.

The first part of the text discusses lower extremity injuries, including commonly seen issues of the foot, ankle, lower leg, knee, hip, and lumbar spine.

The second part of the text discusses upper extremity injuries, including commonly seen issues of the shoulder, elbow, wrist and hand, cervical spine, and head injuries.

Keywords

athletic training, common lower extremity injuries, common upper extremity injuries, concussion, injury prevention, sports medicine

Contents

Preface

Injury Recognition and Prevention: Lower and Upper Extremity is designed for students, coaches, educators and those interested in learning about basic musculoskeletal injuries and conditions that occur in the active population. Each chapter will discuss a different joint and will include a brief review of anatomy, injury recognition, treatment, prevention and provide some rehabilitation guidelines. Injuries are first presented with a brief paragraph allowing for general understanding of the condition. Each injury also provides an associated table which gives the reader a more detailed and concise outline of the condition.

The intent of this text is to serve as a reference tool to give the reader a clear depiction of injuries commonly sustained in the active population. The anatomical joints covered in the text include the foot, ankle, lower leg, knee, hip, lumbar spine, shoulder, elbow, wrist and hand, and cervical spine. Head injuries are discussed as well.

This text is not intended to replace the advice of a physician or other qualified medical professional.

PART I

Lower Extremity

CHAPTER 1

Foot and Toe Injuries

Injuries to the foot and toes are among the most common problems associated with participation in sport. It is essential to understand the basic anatomy of the structures involved in common foot and toe injuries. This chapter describes the anatomy, mechanisms, and common signs and symptoms associated with potential foot and toe conditions.

Anatomy Review

Bone structure (see Figure 1.1):
Forefoot:
Metatarsals and phalanges
Midfoot:
Cuneiforms, cuboid, navicular, LisFranc joint
Rearfoot:
Calcaneus, talus
Tarsals:
1, 2, 3 cuneiforms, cuboid, navicular, talus, calcaneus
Metatarsals:
1 (big toe)–5 (pinky toe)
Phalanges:
Proximal, middle, distal

Musculotendon structure (see Figures 1.2 and 1.3):
Peroneal tendons (longus, brevis, tertius)
Tibialis anterior and posterior
Extensor tendons (digitorum and hallucis)
Flexor tendons (digitorum and hallucis)
Achilles tendon

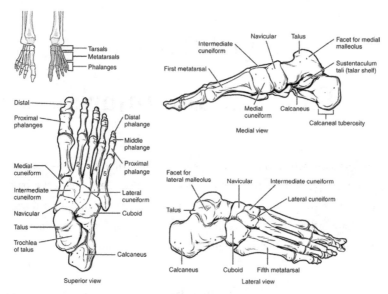

Figure 1.1 Bone anatomy of the foot

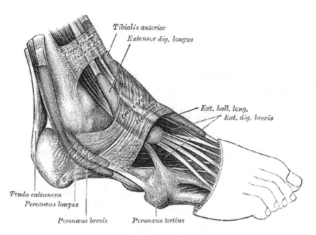

Figure 1.2 Tendons of the foot (lateral view)

Injuries

Pronation and Underpronation

Some of the contributing factors to injuries of the foot include anatomical abnormalities. Two conditions that lend themselves to foot, ankle, and knee problems are both flat feet and high arches. Excessive pronation, or

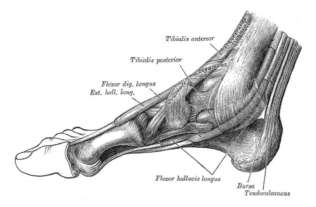

Figure 1.3 Tendons of the foot (medial view)

flat footedness, is marked by an inward roll of the foot. This condition, also referred to as pes planus, is noticeable when the arch collapses while standing or walking. Identification and treatment of this injury are listed in Table 1.1.

Individuals with high arches or underpronation can also be identified by observing the patient both standing and walking. In this situation, the patient presents with an outward roll of the foot, which causes a high arch. The medial arch remains high during both walking and standing, resulting in a condition called pes cavus. Identification and treatment of this injury are listed in Table 1.2.

Table 1.1 Flat foot (pronation and overpronation)

Mechanism of injury	Congenital, weak foot muscles, laxity in foot ligaments
Signs and symptoms	Foot pain, lower leg pain, knee pain, foot falls inward on medial side (see Figure 1.4), shoes broken down on inside
Treatment plan	Medial arch support or orthotics, shoes to limit pronation or increase stability, arch taping
Prevention strategies	Analysis of gait, foot and ankle alignment, proper shoe fitting, strengthening of intrinsic foot muscles

Jones Fracture

Jones fractures occur at the proximal portion of the fifth metatarsal. This location is the most commonly fractured area of the foot because

Table 1.2 High arch (supination and underpronation)

Mechanism of injury	Congenital, tight musculature, tarsals remain rigid during gait
Signs and symptoms	Callus formation on the lateral plantar surface of the foot; shoes broken down on the outside, arch remains high with weight bearing (see Figure 1.4)
Treatment plan	Shoes with more cushion and limit supination or underpronation
Prevention strategies	Analysis of gait, foot and ankle alignment, proper shoe fitting

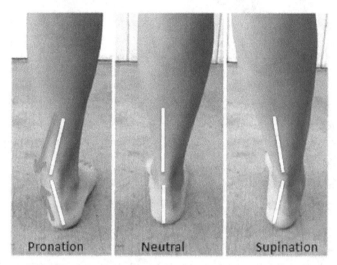

Pronation   Neutral   Supination

Figure 1.4 Pronation/neutral/supination ankle positions

Table 1.3 Jones fracture

Mechanism of injury	Overuse, secondary to an inversion ankle stress, direct blow
Signs and symptoms	Point tender at the styloid process of the fifth metatarsal, pain with or inability to push off during walking
Treatment plan	Walking boot 4–8 weeks, possible surgery
Prevention strategies	Supportive footwear with solid soles

the structural design of the bone makes it inherently unstable. A Jones fracture sometimes results in a nonunion, wherein the fracture does not heal completely due to the lack of good blood supply to the area. A nonunion fracture will require a surgical intervention in order to facilitate healing. Identification and treatment of this injury are listed in Table 1.3.

Corns and Callus

Corns and calluses are caused by constant friction or pressure on specific areas of the foot. Any type of footwear that is ill fitting or too snug may result in blisters to the skin. Over time, the areas where blisters initially formed may turn into rough areas of thickened skin. Calluses generally are flat in appearance and also exhibit a diffused appearance. Corns also consist of thick and rough skin but, compared to calluses, these areas are elevated and smaller in diameter. Corns also tend to be more painful than calluses. Identification and treatment of these conditions are listed in Table 1.4.

Table 1.4 Corns and callus

Mechanism of injury	Friction, loose shoes, not wearing socks
Signs and symptoms	Callus formation, thick rough skin, flaky and dry skin; corns can be tender to pressure
Treatment plan	Elimination of the source of friction, padding, trimming excess skin
Prevention strategies	Well-fitting shoes, wearing two pairs of socks to decrease friction

Bunion

A bunion or hallux valgus occurs when there is excess bone growth at the first metatarsal phalangeal joint. Bunions can be painful and cause gait abnormalities when the great toe is forced toward the second phalanx (hallux valgus). This condition may be congenital, but often occurs in individuals who have worn pointed toe shoes, such as high heels, for a long period of time. In some cases, bunionettes also develop at the fifth metatarsal phalangeal joint. Causes and treatment of bunions and bunionettes are listed in Table 1.5.

Table 1.5 Bunion

Mechanism of injury	Congenital, pressure on the first toe as it is "pushed" laterally, narrow shoes, arthritis
Signs and symptoms	Obvious bump on the joint of the first toe, which grows larger over time, callus formation over the MP joint, first toe deformity—points laterally toward the other toes (hallux valgus). Joint tenderness, decreased range of motion of the first toe

(Continued)

Table 1.5 Bunion (Continued)

Treatment plan	Well-fitting shoes; padding, taping, or splinting; surgical intervention
Prevention strategies	Well-fitting shoes

Morton's Neuroma

Morton's neuroma involves a compression or irritation of the nerves that lie between the metatarsals. This condition most commonly occurs between the third and fourth toes but can occur between others. At-risk populations include people who wear high heels or narrow footwear on a regular basis. This condition can be extremely painful. Identification and treatment of this condition are listed in Table 1.6.

Table 1.6 Morton's neuroma

Mechanism of injury	High-heeled shoes, excess activity on the ball of the foot, narrow shoes
Signs and symptoms	Sharp, burning pain either under the ball of the foot or between the toes. Numbness between the toes
Treatment plan	Supportive shoes, foot pads, decrease impact activity, anti-inflammatory medications. If conservative measures do not work, possible injections or surgery
Prevention strategies	Supportive shoes with wide toe box

Plantar Fasciitis

Plantar fasciitis occurs when there is irritation or inflammation of the plantar fascia located on the undersurface of the foot. The plantar fascia is a thick fibrous band of tissue that serves to support the foot and decrease the amount of stress transmitted up the leg and on other joints. When the plantar fascia is overstretched, tearing of the fascia may occur. This condition is especially painful for individuals who spend a great deal of time on their feet. Often the condition affects one foot, but occasionally it presents bilaterally. Identification and treatment of this condition are listed in Table 1.7.

Table 1.7 Plantar fasciitis

Mechanism of injury	Overuse, overweight, rapid weight gain, forceful landing on foot, forceful push-off, shoes with poor arch support, standing for long periods of time
Signs and symptoms	Sharp, stabbing pain in the bottom of the foot by the heel. Pain with the first steps in the morning that improves as the day goes on. Point tender on the bottom of the foot by the heel, through the arch
Treatment plan	Shoes with good arch support, arch taping, orthotics, ice, massage, stretching of the gastrocnemius muscles and plantar fascia, weight loss, night splint, steroid injections
Prevention strategies	Supportive shoes, maintaining a healthy weight, stretching at the Achilles and foot

Ingrown Toenail

Ingrown toenails are generally the result of the toenail growing into the skin at the side of the nail. This condition is most commonly seen at the big toe and often results in infection. The patient generally presents with pain and swelling surrounding the nail bed that increases with pressure on the affected toe. In order to manage this condition, the ingrown portion of the toenail must be removed and the infection may need to be managed with oral antibiotics, topical antibiotics, or both. More information regarding this condition may be found in Table 1.8.

Table 1.8 Ingrown toenail

Mechanism of injury	Lateral pressure on the corner of the toenail, incorrect toenail cutting, too tight shoes
Signs and symptoms	Pain, redness, and swelling at the corner of the toenail (signs of infection), corner of toenail is imbedded in skin
Treatment plan	Warm soaks, cotton under the toenail, cutting a V into the middle of the nail to help lift the corners out, surgical removal of a portion of the nail, possible antibiotics if signs of infection are present
Prevention strategies	Cutting toenails straight, well-fitting shoes

Turf Toe (First Metatarsal Phalangeal Sprain)

Turf toe involves injury to the soft tissue on the plantar surface of the big toe. More specifically, this condition includes a sprain of the first metatarsophalangeal joint (MTP) and supporting structures. Turf toe is commonly seen in athletes who compete on field turf when an athlete catches his or her big toe on the turf and falls forward. More specific information is listed in Table 1.9.

Table 1.9 Turf toe

Mechanism of injury	Forceful hyperextension, pushing off to run, toe gets stuck on surface, more common on artificial turf, or when using shoes that are too flexible
Signs and symptoms	Pain and swelling at the first MTP joint, pain with pushing off during gait, pain reproduced with hyperflexion of the big toe, limited range of motion, weakness
Treatment plan	Rest, ice, stiff-soled shoes, brace or splint, tape; more severe cases may need a walking boot, toe-strengthening exercises
Prevention strategies	Stiff-soled shoes

Metatarsal Stress Fracture

Metatarsal stress fractures most commonly occur in the second and third metatarsals. Areas of weakness or microfractures of the metatarsals commonly occur when the volume, intensity, or both, of a weight-bearing activity are increased too quickly. These fractures are commonly called "march" fractures, because they are common in military cadets who march in nonsupportive boots. In order to prevent this injury, supportive footwear with good shock absorption is essential, as is a training program that gradually increases volume and intensity of exercise. Identification and treatment of this condition are listed in Table 1.10.

Table 1.10 Metatarsal stress fracture

Mechanism of injury	Repeated microtrauma to the foot, overuse, running, marching, sudden increase in volume or intensity of a weight-bearing exercise
Signs and symptoms	Tenderness or pain at a specific spot on any of the five metatarsals, pain with weight bearing, pain with pushing off, swelling
Treatment plan	Rest, walking boot, activities that are nonweight bearing (swimming, cycling, aqua jogging)
Prevention strategies	Supportive shoes to absorb shock of impact activities and gradual increases in exercise volume and intensity

Fractures of the Phalanges (Toes)

Fractures of the phalanges may occur as a result of stubbing a toe, dropping something on the foot, kicking a hard object, being stepped on, or are the result of a stress fracture that has progressed into a complete break. These mechanisms can cause an incomplete or complete fracture of a phalangeal bone or multiple bones. Toe fractures can be very painful and are hard to manage because the toe is difficult to completely immobilize. Recognition and management of toe fractures are listed in Table 1.11.

Table 1.11 Fractures of the phalanges

Signs and symptoms	Pain at fracture location, pain with weight bearing, swelling of toe, discoloration or bruising of toe, possible deformity
Treatment plan	Rest, walking boot, stiff-soled shoe, activities that are non-weight bearing (swimming, cycling), referral to podiatrist if the toe is deformed
Prevention strategies	Steel-toed shoe if working in a setting where objects may fall on the foot and in other circumstances wearing closed-toe shoes with adequate protection and support

Subungual Hematoma (Blood Under the Nail)

Subungual hematoma formation may occur from being stepped on, wearing shoes that are too small, kicking a hard object, stubbing a toe, or repeated shearing force on the toenail. These mechanisms cause trauma to the nail bed, which results in bleeding and blood pooling under a toenail. In order to reduce pain and relieve pressure, immediate drainage of the hematoma with a drill or cauterization tool is recommended. The patient most likely will lose the nail as it grows out over a period of months. Further recognition and management of subungual hematomas are listed in Table 1.12.

Table 1.12 Subungual hematoma

Signs and symptoms	Blood pooling under the toenail, feeling of pain and pressure under the toenail
Treatment plan	Ice, cauterization or having a hole drilled into the nail to release pressure (should be done in the first 12–48 hours postinjury)
Prevention strategies	Steel-toed shoe if working in a setting where objects may fall on the foot and wearing well-fitting, closed-toe shoes

Lisfranc Injury

A Lisfranc injury involves either a sprain or fracture at the midfoot that disrupts the Lisfranc joint complex. Severity can range from mild to severe. Specifically, Lisfranc injuries occur at the joint complex between the base of the second metatarsal and its interaction with the base of the first and third metatarsals as well as nearby tarsal bones. Besides the bony components of the joint being interrupted, multiple supporting ligaments can be involved. The Lisfranc Joint is an important support structure for the foot and, when injured, is considered a significant injury. Often the Lisfranc joint does not heal properly and a surgical intervention is required to stabilize the joint. Table 1.13 gives specific etiology and treatment for this condition.

Table 1.13 Lisfranc injury

Mechanism of injury	Planting and twisting of the foot, being stepped on, dropped something on the foot, forefoot sprain
Signs and symptoms	Pain and swelling over the midfoot, Lisfranc injuries occur specifically over the base of the second metatarsal Unable to bear weight
Treatment plan	Ice, nonweight bearing, walking boot, referral, possible surgery
Prevention strategies	None

Bibliography

"AAOS—OrthoInfo." n.d. www.orthoinfo.aaos.org/ (accessed January 7, 2016).

Baxter, D.E., D.A. Porter, and L. Schon. 2008. *Baxter's the Foot and Ankle in Sport*. Philadelphia, PA: Mosby Elsevier.

"Diseases and Conditions." n.d. www.mayoclinic.org/diseases-conditions (accessed January 7, 2016).

Joyce, D., and D. Lewindon. 2016. *Sports Injury Prevention and Rehabilitation: Integrating Medicine and Science for Performance Solutions*. New York: Routledge.

Prentice, W.E. 2014. *Principles of Athletic Training: A Competency-Based Approach*. 15th ed. New York: McGraw Hill.

CHAPTER 2

Ankle Injuries

Injuries to the ankle are common within active populations. Because the majority of ankle sprains recur and different structures can be affected with each sprain, it is essential to understand the basic anatomy of the ankle and techniques used to prevent future ankle sprains. This chapter describes the anatomy, mechanisms, and common signs and symptoms associated with ankle injuries. Figures 2.1, 2.2, and 2.3 depict the anatomy of the joint. At the end of the chapter, a basic prevention and rehabilitation program is presented.

Anatomy Review

Bone structure (see Figure 2.1):
    Tarsals:
        Talus, calcaneus
    Fibula:
        Lateral malleolus
    Tibia:
        Medial malleolus

Ligamentous structure (see Figure 2.1):
    Anterior talofibular ligament
    Calcaneofibular ligament
    Posterior talofibular ligament
    Anterior inferior tibiofibular ligament
    Posterior inferior tibiofibular ligament
    Deltoid ligaments (4 bands, medial side)

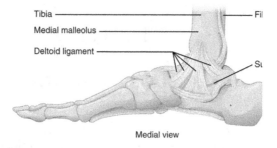

Tibia ———————
Medial malleolus ———————
Deltoid ligament ———————
Fil
Sι

Medial view

Fibula ———
Interosseous membrane
Tibia
Posterior and anterior inferiσ tibiofibular ligaments
Anterior talofibular ligament

Calcaneofibular ligament   Subtalar joint

Lateral view

Figure 2.1 Ligaments of the ankle

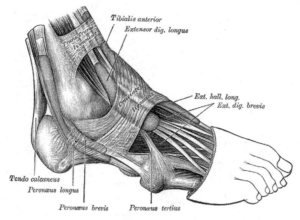

Tibialis anterior
Extensor dig. longus

Ext. hall. long.
Ext. dig. brevis

Tendo calcaneus
Peronæus longus
Peronæus brevis   Peronæus tertius

Figure 2.2 Tendons of the ankle (lateral view)

Musculotendon structure (see Figures 2.2 and 2.3):
    Peroneal tendons (longus, brevis, tertius)
    Tibialis anterior and posterior

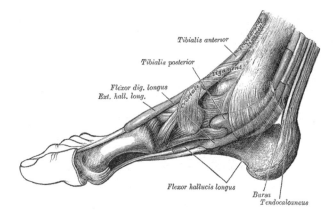

Figure 2.3 Tendons of the ankle (medial view)

Extensor tendons (digitorum and hallucis)
Flexor tendons (digitorum and hallucis)
Achilles tendon

Injuries

Lateral Ankle Sprain (Inversion Stress)

The majority of all ankle sprains occur as a result of inversion stress. Lateral ankle sprains occur when the ankle is "rolled in," causing a stretching of the structures on the outside of the ankle while concurrently, the structures on the medial side (inside) of the ankle sustain a compression force. Ankle sprains can range in severity from a first degree to a third degree sprain and can involve one ligament or multiple ligaments, including the anterior talofibular ligament, the calcaneofibular ligament, or the posterior talofibular ligament. The severity of the sprain can be described by the extent of injury to one of these ligaments on the lateral side or by the number of ligaments involved. The more ligaments involved, the more severe the sprain. Additional anatomical structures on the lateral side of the ankle can also incur damage when inversion stress occurs, including straining the peroneal muscles, possibly fracturing the styloid process of the fifth metatarsal or sustaining a contusion to the compressed medial

Table 2.1 Lateral ankle sprain

Mechanism of injury	Inversion stress, rolling the ankle inwards as a result of inappropriate landings, trail running, stepping in a pothole, falling off a curb
Signs and symptoms	Pain and swelling around the lateral ankle, discoloration or bruising around the joint
Treatment plan	Ice, decreased range of motion, maintaining the joint in a 90° neutral position, using compression bandage, possible nonweight bearing depending on severity, strengthening the ankle muscles, balance training, taping, or bracing
Prevention strategies	Strengthening of muscles around the ankle, balance exercises, bracing or taping

anatomical structures. Mechanism, signs and symptoms, and management of this injury are listed in Table 2.1.

Medial Ankle Sprain (Eversion Stress)

A medial or eversion ankle sprain is more commonly known as a deltoid ligament sprain. There are four deltoid ligaments that support the ankle on the medial side. Sprains to these ligaments are less common than those to the lateral ankle. Damage to the ligaments can range from mild to severe and are graded as first, second, or third degree sprains, respectively. When the ankle is excessively and forcefully rolled outward, or everted, there is considerable stress placed on the medial aspect of the joint. This injury can occur as a result of unexpected changes in direction, such as stepping into a pothole, falling off a curb, or rapid, unplanned changes in velocity and momentum. Table 2.2 describes signs, symptoms, and management of this injury.

High Ankle Sprain (Syndesmosis)

Spraining the proximal ligaments of the lateral ankle, which includes the anterior inferior tibiofibular ligament and the posterior inferior tibiofibular ligament, is less common but generally take longer to heal than a typical lateral ankle sprain. It is not uncommon for the syndesmotic space above the joint line to separate, which will add another level

Table 2.2 Medial ankle sprain

Signs and symptoms	Pain and swelling around the medial ankle, discoloration or bruising around the joint, could also present with pain on the lateral side from the bones bruising, unable to bear weight
Treatment plan	Ice, decreased range of motion, maintaining the joint in a 90° neutral position, using compression bandage, possible nonweight bearing depending on severity, strengthening the ankle muscles, balance training, taping, or bracing
Prevention strategies	Strengthening of muscles around the ankle, balance exercises, bracing or taping

Table 2.3 High ankle sprain

Mechanism of injury	Inversion stress with rotational force, hyperdorsiflexion of the ankle, such as jumping from a tall structure or planting and rotating the ankle
Signs and symptoms	Pain and swelling high around the lateral ankle and close to the tibiofibular joint; pain or inability to weight bear, pain with push off
Treatment plan	Ice, nonweight bearing, walking boot, possible surgery if disruption of the joint cannot be resolved with conservative treatment. Rehabilitation is the same as a lateral ankle sprain, taping, bracing
Prevention strategies	Strengthening of muscles around the ankle, balance exercises, bracing or taping

of disability. Signs and symptoms and management of this injury are listed in Table 2.3.

Achilles Tendon Injury (Strain or Rupture)

The Achilles tendon connects the gastrocnemius and soleus muscles to the calcaneus bone of the foot. Acute and chronic injury to this tendon is common and can range in severity from mild acute strains, to chronic tendon irritation, and even full rupture of the tendon. Injury to the tendon almost always results in pain at the back of the ankle. Achilles tendon strains are most common in athletes who repetitively run or jump, while complete rupture of the Achilles tendon generally happens in middle-aged

Table 2.4 Achilles tendon injury

Mechanism of injury	*Strain:* Overuse with running, excessive dorsiflexion *Rupture:* Forceful push-off against resistance
Signs and symptoms	*Strain:* Tenderness along the Achilles tendon, can occur acutely or gradually; swelling behind the ankle; pain while climbing stairs, walking, running; weakness *Rupture:* A snap or pop is felt or heard. Patients may state that it "felt like they have been kicked or shot in the back of the ankle" Swelling, pain behind the ankle, or inability to do a toe raise
Treatment plan	*Strain:* Ice, taping, anti-inflammatory medications, stretching, strengthening *Rupture:* Ice, crutches, rest, referral to orthopedic surgeon for assessment of conservative treatment versus surgical intervention
Prevention strategies	Stretching of the gastrocnemius and soleus muscle complex

adults. This is known as a "weekend warrior" injury because it usually occurs to those who participate in adult sporting leagues. A full rupture may require up to nine months of rehabilitation. More information regarding the cause and treatment of this condition is listed in Table 2.4.

Prevention and Rehabilitation of General Ankle Injuries

The following rehabilitation exercises may be used in order to achieve full range of motion and strengthen the structures in the ankle to prevent initial or future injury. These exercises may also be used postinjury to regain range of motion, strength, and neuromuscular control. Muscles targeted during the rehabilitation process are shown in Figures 2.4 and 2.5.

A. *Maintaining and reestablishing range of motion*:
   a. Achieving or maintaining joint flexibility is an important aspect of injury prevention. After an ankle injury, regaining movement is an important part of the rehabilitation process and the ability to return to normal activities.

b. Range-of-motion exercises can be progressive in nature, starting with small movements and working up to large movements

c. Exercise options include:

    i. abc's—drawing the alphabet with your big toe serving as the "pencil"

    ii. Ankle pumps—plantarflexion, dorsiflexion, inversion, and eversion

    iii. Ankle circles—smaller circles gradually getting larger

    iv. Gastrocnemius and soleus stretching using a towel or band to pull the foot toward the body

d. All stretches should be held for 20 to 30 seconds and repeated two to three times bilaterally

B. *Maintaining and reestablishing strength*:

a. Increasing the strength of the muscles around the ankle and lower leg will help provide support to the ligaments and ankle joint and prevent future injuries.

b. Muscles to be targeted include:

    i. Gastrocnemius and soleus complex (plantarflexion): see Figure 2.4

    ii. Anterior tibialis (dorsiflexion): see Figure 2.4

    iii. Peroneals (eversion): see Figure 2.5

    iv. Posterior tibialis (plantarflexion and inversion): see Figure 2.5

c. Progression: Initially exercises can be performed using no weight and then can be performed using ankle weights or resistance bands.

d. Volume, frequency, and duration: A basic rehabilitation protocol generally includes three sets of 10 repetitions for each exercise, three times per week for four to eight weeks.

C. *Maintaining or reestablishing balance*:

1. Progressive sequence of balance exercises easiest (a) to most difficult (c):

a. One-legged stance on a flat surface

b. One-legged stance on a flat surface with eyes closed

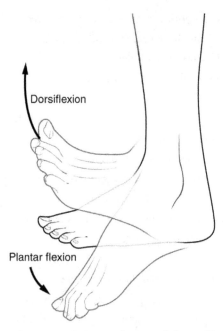

Figure 2.4 Dorsiflexion and plantarflexion of the ankle

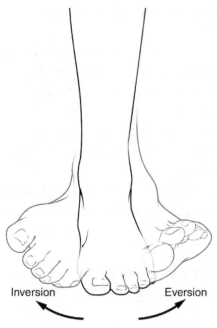

Figure 2.5 Inversion and eversion of the ankle

    c. One-legged stance on an uneven surface (pillow, mini trampoline, etc.)

2. Begin the balance program using exercise (a). Each balance exercise should initially be performed for 30 seconds on each leg and progressively increase in duration until the task seems easy. Once the task has been mastered on both sides, progress to the next exercise.

Bibliography

"AAOS—OrthoInfo." n.d. www.orthoinfo.aaos.org/ (accessed January 7, 2016).

Baxter, D.E., D.A. Porter, and L. Schon. 2008. *Baxter's the Foot and Ankle in Sport*. Philadelphia, PA: Mosby Elsevier.

"Diseases and Conditions." n.d. www.mayoclinic.org/diseases-conditions (accessed January 7, 2016).

Houglum, P.A. 2010. *Therapeutic Exercise for Musculoskeletal Injuries*. Champaign, IL: Human Kinetics.

CHAPTER 3

Lower Leg Injuries

Injuries to the lower leg can be complex in nature because numerous anatomical structures can be involved. In addition to the bony anatomy, the lower leg is separated into four "compartments," wherein all of the musculature, nerves, and blood vessels are housed. Injuries to the lower leg vary in severity depending on the mechanism and structures involved. The following chapter introduces basic anatomy of and common sport injuries to the lower leg. Also outlined for each injury are: signs and symptoms, treatment and rehabilitation, and prevention strategies.

Anatomy Review

Bone structure (see Figure 3.1):

Fibula:

Head of the fibula, lateral malleolus

Tibia:

Tibial tuberosity, pes anserine, Gerdy's tubercle, plateau, medial malleolus

Ligamentous structure:

Anterior superior tibiofibular ligament

Posterior superior tibiofibular ligament

Anterior inferior tibiofibular ligament

Posterior inferior tibiofibular ligament

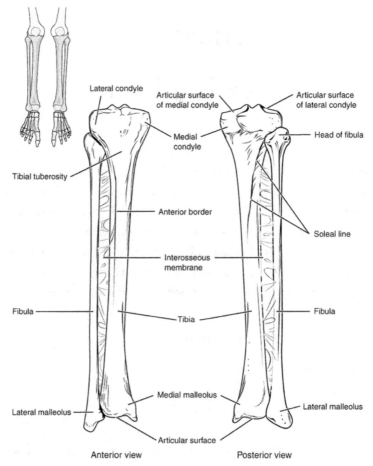

Figure 3.1 Bone anatomy of the low leg

Compartments of lower leg and contents (see Figure 3.2):

A. *Anterior compartment*

1. Tibialis anterior
2. Extensor hallucis longus
3. Extensor digitorum longus
4. Peroneus tertius
5. Deep peroneal nerve
6. Anterior tibial artery

B. *Lateral compartment*

    1. Peroneus longus

    2. Peroneus brevis

    3. Superficial peroneal nerve

C. *Superficial posterior compartment*

    1. Gastrocnemius

    2. Soleus

    3. Plantaris tendon

D. *Deep posterior compartment*

    1. Tibialis posterior

    2. Flexor digitorum longus

    3. Flexor hallucis longus

    4. Posterior tibial artery

    5. Peroneal artery

    6. Posterior tibial nerve

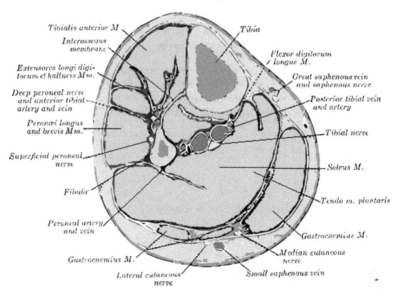

Figure 3.2 **Compartments of the low leg (cross-section view)**

Injuries

Medial Tibial Stress Syndrome (Shin Splints)

Medial tibial stress syndrome, MTSS (also known as: shin splints), is a common exercise-related injury that occurs in the low leg. Pain occurs usually after increases in volume or intensity of physical activity, especially running. MTSS is a progressive condition that usually starts with a muscle strain and progresses to irritation of the lining of the bone and can result in a stress reaction, typically along the tibia. MTSS can also involve the anterior or posterior tibialis muscles. This condition is commonly seen in individuals with poor foot mechanics, improper footwear, or lack of training and conditioning. Table 3.1 identifies mechanisms, signs and symptoms, and treatment of MTSS.

Table 3.1 Medial tibial stress syndrome

Mechanism of injury	Flat feet or pronation, wearing worn-out shoes, wearing flip-flops, overuse, running on hard surfaces, sudden increases in activity level
Signs and symptoms	Progression of pain and its location: starting in the muscles of the low leg, moving to pain along the medial border of the tibia (broad area of pain) and progressing to pain at a focal point on the tibia (stress reaction). Muscle weakness, pain that is present over a progressively longer time (during activity, after activity, pain all the time)
Treatment plan	Ice, stretching, arch support (new shoes or taping), biomechanical evaluation, changing running surface, nonweight-bearing activities (swimming, cycling, elliptical exercise machines)
Prevention strategies	Slow progression of volume and intensity of running, supportive shoes, arch taping, stretching

Compartment Syndrome (Acute or Chronic)

Compartment syndrome is a serious condition that can occur in any of the four lower leg compartments but most commonly occurs in the anterior and lateral compartments. Each compartment in the lower leg is separated by fascia and contains muscles, arteries, veins, and nerves.

Table 3.2 Compartment syndrome

Mechanism of injury	Chronic: overuse, running, common in people who run on their toes Acute: direct blow to the lower leg, fracture of the tibia or fibula, severe high ankle sprain
Signs and symptoms	Chronic: pressure pain, pain in entire compartment, pain decreases with cessation of the activity, foot "falls asleep" during activity but returns to normal with cessation of activity Acute: severe pain, pressure feeling, leg feels hard, shiny appearance to the skin, weak muscles in the compartment, numb foot, decreased circulation in foot
Treatment plan	Chronic: stretching muscles within the compartment, identifying any existing biomechanical problems, possible surgical intervention if conservative treatment is not successful Acute: immediate referral to an orthopedic surgeon to release pressure in the compartment
Prevention strategies	Maintain flexibility in lower leg muscles, supportive shoes

Compartment syndrome results when the space inside a compartment becomes compromised and the vascular and nervous structures within it are compressed. Compartment syndrome can occur gradually over time or can occur acutely in conjunction with lower leg fractures or trauma. Acute compartment syndrome is considered a medical emergency. Long-term compression of vascular and nervous structures within the lower leg can have detrimental effects on the foot, including numbness, tingling, and loss of function. Identification and treatment information for this condition is identified in Table 3.2.

Deep Vein Thrombophlebitis

Deep vein thrombophlebitis (DVT) occurs when a clot forms deep within the venous system, most commonly in the veins of the legs. This is typically the result of prolonged bed rest, sitting for extended periods of time, or immobilization due to surgery or injury. DVT is more likely to occur in older individuals but has been reported in younger populations as well. Life threatening complications, such as blood clots, or pulmonary embolism could occur if DVT is left untreated. Further explanation of DVT is listed in Table 3.3.

Table 3.3 Deep vein thrombophlebitis

Mechanism of injury	Sitting for long periods of time, long flights or drives, postsurgical immobilization, prolonged bed rest
Signs and symptoms	Leg pain, muscle soreness—usually calf, whole-leg swelling, can occur without symptoms as well, Imaging the lower extremities is almost always used for diagnosis
Treatment plan	Prescription blood thinners (under a medical doctor's care)
Prevention strategies	Frequent movement, especially on long flights or drives, improving range of motion early postsurgery, muscle pumping exercises, wearing compression stockings, daily aspirin

Tibia or Fibula Fracture

Fractures of the tibia and fibula can occur individually or simultaneously. The tibia serves to bear the majority of body weight of the low leg, whereas the fibula acts as an accessory bone that also forms the lateral portion of the ankle. Complicated fractures of the tibia, fibula, or both, are often the result of direct trauma and require surgical intervention, including plates or screws to reconstruct the bony structures. More information regarding these fractures is listed in Table 3.4.

Table 3.4 Tibia or fibula fracture

Mechanism of injury	Direct blow, progression of a stress fracture, falling from a height, car accident
Signs and symptoms	Point tender in one specific location on the bone, deformity, swelling, inability to bear weight, broken leg may appear shorter or rotated
Treatment plan	Referral to an orthopedic surgeon, crutches, rest, ice, muscle strengthening
Prevention strategies	Wear protective equipment

Bibliography

"AAOS—OrthoInfo." n.d. www.orthoinfo.aaos.org/ (accessed January 7, 2016).

"Diseases and Conditions." n.d. www.mayoclinic.org/diseases-conditions (accessed January 7, 2016).

Prentice, W.E. 2014. *Principles of Athletic Training: A Competency-Based Approach.* New York: McGraw Hill.

Rome, K., and P. McNair. 2015. *Management of Chronic Conditions in the Foot and Lower Leg.* Edinburgh: Churchill Livingstone.

CHAPTER 4

Knee Injuries

The knee joint is the largest joint in the body and is vital for mobility and most activities that involve the lower body. The structure of the knee is made sound by the ligaments and muscles that originate at the femur, move across the knee, and insert distally at the tibia and fibula. These structures help to stabilize the knee joint but still leave the surrounding area vulnerable to injury. Chronic repetitive motions of the knee, contact sports, sports that require quick directional changes, or landing on a hard surface, all challenge this somewhat fragile musculoskeletal structure. Knee injuries are common and can have a great impact on a person's ability to perform activities of daily living and athletic performance. This chapter outlines common knee injuries as well as signs and symptoms, treatments, and prevention techniques.

Anatomy Review

Bone structure (see Figure 4.1):

Femur:

> Femoral condyles, epicondyles, intercondylar notch or fossa, patellar groove, adductor tubercle

Tibia:

> Tibial plateau, tibial tuberosity, Gerdy's tubercle, pes anserine

Fibula:

> Head

Patella:

> Large sesamoid bone, should slide smoothly in femoral groove, articular facets, and cartilage

Ligamentous structure (see Figure 4.1):

Anterior cruciate ligament (ACL)

Prevents anterior translation of the tibia on the femur

Posterior cruciate ligament (PCL)

Prevents posterior translation of the tibia on the femur

Medial collateral ligament (MCL)

Prevents valgus translation of tibia

Lateral collateral ligament (LCL)

Prevents varus translation of tibia

Musculotendon structure (see Figure 4.1):

Suprapatellar tendon—engulfs the patella, attaches to patella

Infrapatellar tendon (patellar tendon)—also referred to as the patellar ligament

Rectus femoris—most superficial quadricep muscle

Vastus medialis, lateralis, and intermedius—additional quadricep muscles

Semitendinosus, gracilis, sartorius

Iliotibial band (IT)—attaches tensor fascia latae and gluteus maximus to Gerdy's tubercle

Semimembranosus and semitendinosus (medial hamstrings)

Biceps femoris (lateral hamstring)

Gastrocnemius and soleus

Other anatomical structure (see Figure 4.1):

Meniscus

Medial—(C shaped)

Lateral—(O shaped)

Bursae

Prepatellar bursae

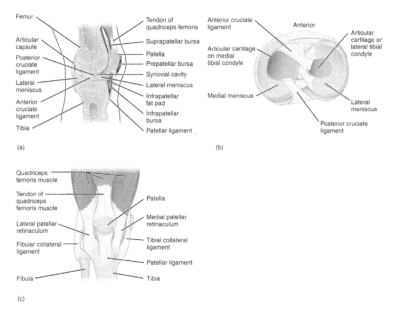

Figure 4.1 **Anatomy of the knee: (a) sagittal section through the right knee joint; (b) superior view of the right tibia in the knee joint, showing the menisci and cruciate ligaments; and (c) anterior view of right knee**

Injuries

MCL Sprain

The MCL is found on the medial side or "inside" of the knee, and connects the femur to the tibia. The MCL helps prevent valgus stress, which can be created by a blow to the knee from the outside and is the most commonly injured ligament of the knee. Sprains to the MCL can be graded from first to third degree. The MCL is composed of two bands of tissue, and injury to the deeper band of the MCL can result in damage to the medial meniscus because some of its fibers insert into the cartilaginous structure. When stress testing for damage, the MCL is best isolated at 20° to 30° of flexion and the majority of pain will be noted at the end of full extension and full flexion of the knee. The mechanism of injury and management of this condition may be found in Table 4.1.

Table 4.1 MCL sprain

Mechanism of injury	Valgus force (direct blow to the lateral side of the knee): with or without twisting
Signs and symptoms	Point tender over the MCL, point tender over the origin and insertion of the ligament, swelling, knee feeling unstable, pain with full extension or full flexion of the knee
Treatment plan	Ice, brace 4–6 weeks, avoid terminal extension and full flexion initially; surgical intervention is typically not needed unless the meniscus is involved, rehabilitation (range of motion and strength)
Prevention strategies	Muscle strengthening, protective bracing to prevent collateral force

LCL Sprain

The LCL is found on the outside, or lateral side, of the knee and connects the femur to the fibula. It is more cord-like in structure and better protected, thus is less commonly injured compared to the other ligaments. Injury to the LCL involves a blow to the knee from the inside of the knee, which is also a less common mechanism. LCL injuries are most commonly seen in wrestlers or in knee injuries that are all encompassing. The LCL is also more elastic and thus more resilient to stress. Management strategies for this injury may be found in Table 4.2.

Table 4.2 LCL sprain

Mechanism of injury	Varus stress (direct blow from the medial side of the knee)
Signs and symptoms	Pain at the head of the fibula and over LCL, swelling, knee feeling unstable
Treatment plan	Ice, heals quickly, 2–4 weeks, evaluate postlateral structures of the knee that could also be involved
Prevention strategies	Muscle strengthening, protective bracing to prevent collateral force

ACL Sprain

A sprain of the ACL is the second most common ligament injury to the knee. Sports that involve a lot of directional change (football, basketball, and soccer) typically see a high rate of ACL injuries, but ACL sprains can occur within any sport. ACL sprains are also more common in females than males; a variety of hypotheses exist to explain this phenomenon and include the following: decreased fitness levels, muscular imbalance, decreased neuromuscular control, improper landing biomechanics or all of these; differences in hip and lower extremity alignment; laxity of ligaments; and estrogen-induced increases in ligament mobility.

The ACL sits deep in the knee joint in a diagonal direction and forms a cross with the PCL, hence its "cruciate" name. It prevents anterior translation of the tibia on the femur and also serves as a pivot for the knee when reaching terminal extension. Damage to other structures of the knee are common when an ACL injury occurs, especially articular cartilage, the meniscus, and other ligaments, which can make the injury more complex. Partial tears to the ACL are not as common as complete tears; therefore, the ACL typically requires surgical reconstruction, especially if an athlete wishes to return to sport. Playing with an ACL-deficient knee increases risk of further injury to the meniscus and articular cartilage. Signs and symptoms of this injury and management strategies are listed in Table 4.3.

Table 4.3 ACL sprain

Mechanism of injury	Hyperextension of the knee, planting the foot and twisting the knee, deceleration, changing directions quickly, improper landing from a jump, direct blow
Signs and symptoms	Immediate sharp pain that dissipates, hearing or feeling a "pop," involuntary cessation of activity, anterior pain, posterior pain, (sometimes no pain), significant joint swelling within minutes to hours, instability of the joint (falling to one side)
Treatment plan	Usually reconstructive surgery followed by about 6 to 9+ months of rehabilitation, which emphasizes range of motion and quad and hamstring strength to protect the new ligament
Prevention strategies	Increase in hip and knee strength, functional training activities using multiple planes of motion

PCL Sprain

The PCL sits deep in the knee behind the ACL, making the back portion of the "cross." It prevents posterior tibial translation on the femur and is less commonly injured than the other ligaments around the knee. Injury to the PCL occurs when the tibia is forced posteriorly, usually with a bent knee. Examples of scenarios in which this injury may occur include: landing hard on the ground with the knee(s) bent, or in the event of a car accident in which the knees hit the dashboard. Hyperextension of the knee is another PCL injury mechanism. Additional information regarding PCL injuries can be found in Table 4.4.

Table 4.4 PCL sprain

Signs and symptoms	Immediate posterior pain, swelling that comes on quickly within minutes to hours, instability
Treatment plan	Ice, heals rapidly if it is the only structure involved, brace, rehabilitation emphasizing range of motion and quadricep strengthening
Prevention strategies	Quad and hamstring strengthening. Functional training activities using multiple planes of motion

Meniscus Tears

The menisci are wedge-shaped structures that sit on top of the tibial plateau and are important to the structure and function of the knee. The menisci also provide stability and cushion between the femur and tibia as well as protect the hyaline cartilage on the surfaces of the tibia and femur. Meniscus tears are among the most common knee injuries and can occur as a result of many different mechanisms. Generally, meniscal tears are described by the shape and location of the injury. When describing injury location, the meniscus is often divided into three zones based on the amount of blood flow to each region. Tears that occur to the outer zone of the meniscus wedge typically have better blood supply and tend to heal more quickly and completely. Tears that occur to the inner zone generally need surgical intervention because there is little to no blood supply to facilitate healing. Further information regarding meniscal tears is located in Table 4.5.

Table 4.5 Meniscal tears

Mechanism of injury	Deep squats (repeated or acute), planting the foot and twisting the knee, degeneration of the meniscal tissue with age
Signs and symptoms	Pain along the joint line; effusion possible; catching, locking, clicking, or popping sensations; unstable; giving out; feeling like pressure in the knee; pain with walking up or down stairs or squatting; unable to move knee through the full range of motion
Treatment plan	Ice, rehabilitation, possibly crutches, anti-inflammatory medications Peripheral (outer rim) tears typically require surgical repair Central tears (inner rim) typically require surgical removal
Prevention strategies	Maintain a healthy weight, avoid deep squat activities, strengthening of the quadriceps

Prepatellar Bursitis

Bursae are fluid-filled sacs located all over the body, especially in joint areas between bony prominences and tendons or other soft tissues. Bursae serve a protective role, provide cushioning, and prevent friction. In the event the bursa becomes irritated, usually as a result of repetitive motion or a direct blow, it can fill with fluid and decrease the mobility of the surrounding structures. The most commonly injured bursa in the knee is the prepatellar bursa, which sits on top of the patella. Irritation to the prepatellar bursa is common in sports in which the athlete has the potential to take a hit to the knee (turf, wood floor, ice, opponent, etc.). A bursitis can be uncomfortable and can limit the patient's range of motion but usually resolves without lasting debilitation. Management of this injury is detailed in Table 4.6.

Table 4.6 Prepatellar bursitis

Mechanism of injury	Direct blow, kneeling for long periods of time, rheumatoid arthritis, gout, infection
Signs and symptoms	Rapid swelling of the bursa presenting with a distinct goose egg shape over the patella, movement may be limited due to the amount of fluid, typically pain free unless the injury is a direct blow
Treatment plan	Ice, compression, activity as tolerated, anti-inflammatory medications, draining of the bursa, surgical removal if chronic
Prevention strategies	Wear knee pads, avoid repetitive kneeling by sitting on a stool

IT Band Friction Syndrome

Iliotibial band friction syndrome (ITBS) occurs on the lateral and outside of the knee where the IT band extends over bony prominences of the femur. The IT band runs from the hip to the knee and provides stability to the lateral aspect of the knee during running. Friction of the band over bony prominences commonly occurs in sports with repetitive leg motions like running, biking, and repetitive squatting, and can cause lateral knee pain. Management of this condition is addressed in Table 4.7.

Table 4.7 IT band friction syndrome

Mechanism of injury	Overuse, running, biking, repetitive squatting motion, running on a banked street or track in the same direction, breaststroke in swimming, rowing Other causes: leg length difference, poor shoe support, increased mileage, hill work, weak hip abductors, overpronation
Signs and symptoms	Pain on the lateral femoral epicondyle, pain can be felt during activity and as the syndrome progresses, pain will become more constant, pain is felt during foot strike, tight hamstrings, and IT band
Treatment plan	Address the initial cause of the injury, neutralize pronation, stretch hamstrings and IT band, ice, ultrasound, massage, rest or reduction in activity
Prevention strategies	Proper shoes, stretching of the IT band, strengthening of the hip abductors, alternating directions on a track or road when running

Osgood Schlatter Disease

Osgood Schlatter disease presents with pain and a lump on the front of the knee at the tibial tuberosity; specifically, the pain is over a traction growth plate where the quadricep tendon pulls on its attachment site on the tibia. It most often occurs in children who play sports such as basketball, running, dance, and soccer or another type of activity that involves a lot of jumping and changing of direction. Osgood Schlatter seems to be more common in boys and typically occurs between the ages of 11 and 14 years. Once the patient has reached his or her adult height, the pain diminishes but the visible bump remains. More information regarding this condition may be found in Table 4.8.

Table 4.8 Osgood Schlatter disease

Mechanism of injury	Rapid growth in conjunction with potential overuse of the knee joint, repetitive jumping activities and running
Signs and symptoms	Point tender over tibial tuberosity especially with running and jumping, tibial tuberosity may protrude, pain with quadricep muscle testing
Treatment plan	Rest, ice, decrease activity until pain has diminished, Cho-Pat strap, strengthen the quadriceps
Prevention strategies	N/A

Patellar Tendinopathy

Patellar Tendinopathy, also known as "jumper's knee," is painful inflammation of the patellar tendon, which serves to connect the quadricep muscles to the tibia by running over and engulfing the patella. Tendinopathy is a common condition, as tendons can be aggravated by repetitive activity. The patellar tendon is especially susceptible to inflammation as a result of repetitive jumping and running and is a common injury among basketball and volleyball athletes. Tendinopathy can be acute or chronic; in either instance, pain management is key to minimizing loss of playing time. There are many methods of treatment for this condition and further information regarding patellar tendinopathy can be located in Table 4.9.

Table 4.9 Patellar tendinopathy

Signs and symptoms	Point tender over the middle or attachment points of the patellar tendon, feels better after warm-up, crepitus, pain with climbing and descending stairs, tight hamstrings and quadriceps, muscle imbalance
Treatment plan	Rest, decrease inflammation via ice, ultrasound, anti-inflammatory medications stretch the quadriceps and hamstrings, strengthen the muscles around the knee, address biomechanical issues, Cho-Pat strap
Prevention strategies	Quadricep and hamstring strengthening. Increase vastus medialis oblique strength. Alternate training surfaces between hard and soft surfaces

Patellar Dislocation and Subluxation

Patellar dislocations occur when the patella slides out of the patellar groove of the femur and remains in this abnormal position. The dislocation typically occurs in the lateral direction and is more common in sports such as football, soccer, basketball, and hockey. Several factors could predispose athletes to dislocations of the patella, including muscle imbalance (tight lateral structures, weak medial structures) and large Q angles (wider hips, knocked knees, and pronated feet).

Patellar subluxations occur when the patella slips out of its normal alignment but slides back into place on its own. This injury can also be referred to as patellar instability. Both of these conditions can occur due to pivoting on a straight leg, strong quadricep contractions, direct blow, or sudden change in direction. Table 4.10 further describes management of this condition.

Table 4.10 Patellar dislocation and subluxation

Signs and symptoms	*Dislocation*: severe pain, flexed knee, deformity with the patella sitting on the lateral side of the joint, swelling *Subluxation*: pain, sensation of the knee giving out, pop, or click
Treatment plan	Straighten knee along with slight medial pressure on the patella to reduce the dislocation, ice, brace, rehabilitation including strengthening of medial quadricep and stretching of lateral structures, possible lateral retinaculum release if conservative treatment does not work
Prevention strategies	Maintain muscle balance between the medial and lateral quadriceps, stretching of the IT band

Quadriceps Tendon Mechanical Rupture

The quadriceps tendon is formed by the combination of the quadriceps muscles just above the patella before it continues down the front of the knee to the patellar tendon. A complete tear of this tendon above the patella is more common in middle-aged people during running or jumping activities. This is a traumatic injury that causes immediate disability. Common mechanisms are: a direct blow to a flexed quadriceps, awkward jump landing, or having a large force placed on the leg with a bent knee. Further information regarding quadriceps tendon ruptures can be located in Table 4.11.

Table 4.11 Quadriceps tendon mechanical rupture

Signs and symptoms	Pain, swelling, feeling a pop, feeling a tearing sensation, visible or palpable indentation above the patella, patella might sag, inability to extend the leg, instability
Treatment plan	Ice, immobilization, referral for surgical repair, anti-inflammatory medications, strengthening
Prevention strategies	N/A

Chondromalacia

Chondromalacia is the general term for the breakdown or degeneration of the cartilage under the patella, and can also be known as patellofemoral pain syndrome. Chondromalacia pain can increase with age and is more common in females and active adults who have participated in running or jumping activities. Generally, this condition results from overuse, unbalanced quadricep muscle strength, previous patellar injuries, sudden increases in activity volume or intensity or both, and weak hip abductors. More information regarding this condition may be found in Table 4.12.

Table 4.12 Chondromalacia

Signs and symptoms	Dull, achy patellofemoral pain especially with walking up or down stairs, terminal extension of the knee causes pain, pushing the patella into the patellar groove recreates the pain, pain with squatting, knee may be stiff or sore after sitting for long periods of time
Treatment plan	Treat pain, rest, ice, anti-inflammatory medications. Find mechanical cause such as muscle imbalance that puts uneven pressure on the patella, cross-training
Prevention strategies	Activities that create less stress on the knees such as biking and swimming, loss of excess weight, stretching

Tibial Plateau Fracture

The tibial plateau is the superior portion of the tibia that forms the inferior portion of the knee joint and houses the meniscus. A fracture of this portion of the tibia is considered a severe injury because the fracture can also cause damage to other tissues including blood vessels, nerves, and cartilage. A fracture occurs typically as a result of a traumatic force but may be a continuation of a stress reaction to the top of tibia. Typically, surgery will be needed to restore the anatomical structure of the knee. Fractures to the tibial plateau result from violent valgus or varus stress to the knee. A direct blow, fall from a height, or motor vehicle accident can also be mechanisms of injury. Table 4.13 further describes the management of this condition.

Table 4.13 Tibial plateau fracture

Signs and symptoms	Leg or joint deformity, severe pain, unable to bear weight, swelling, cold feeling foot, numbness
Treatment plan	Referral, crutches, possible surgery dependent on severity and type of fracture, regain range of motion and strength
Prevention strategies	N/A

Osteochondritis Dissecans

Osteochondritis dissecans (OCD), also known as avascular necrosis of the femoral condyle, occurs when the bone under the articular cartilage dies due to localized circulation impairment and subsequent necrosis. This injury can be further complicated if pieces of bone tissue become loose and lodged within the joint space. This condition can also potentially lead to early-onset osteoarthritis. Although OCD lesions can occur in multiple joints, young athletes most commonly experience this condition in the knee due to participation in high impact sports. Mechanisms associated with this condition include repetitive impact injury and possibly genetics. Additional information regarding this condition is listed in Table 4.14.

Table 4.14 Osteochondritis dissecans

Signs and symptoms	Gradual onset of pain, swelling after activity, clicking or catching if loose fragment involved, point tender over femoral condyle
Treatment plan	Referral to a medical doctor, possible surgery followed by rehabilitation
Prevention strategies	N/A

Popliteal Cyst

Also known as a Baker's cyst, popliteal cysts occur when there is a herniation of excess fluid from within the knee that bulges out behind the knee. The cyst is caused by previous injury within the knee joint; therefore, determining the underlying cause is the most important aspect of the treatment plan. This condition may be associated with a meniscus tear or arthritic conditions. Management strategies are listed in Table 4.15.

Table 4.15 Popliteal cyst

Signs and symptoms	Visible and palpable fluid-filled cyst behind the knee, decreased range of motion, knee stiffness, pain, symptoms increase after activity
Treatment plan	Determine the underlying cause and treat accordingly, restrict activity to pain free movement, compression sleeve
Prevention strategies	Proper treatment of initial injury to avoid recurrence

Bibliography

"AAOS—OrthoInfo." n.d. www.orthoinfo.aaos.org/ (accessed January 7, 2016).

"Diseases and Conditions." n.d. www.mayoclinic.org/diseases-conditions (accessed January 7, 2016).

Prentice, W.E. 2014. *Principles of Athletic Training: A Competency-Based Approach.* New York: McGraw Hill.

Rodríguez-Merchán, E.C. 2013. *Traumatic Injuries of the Knee.* Milan, Italy: Springer.

CHAPTER 5

Hip and Thigh Injuries

The hip is a ball-and-socket joint, which allows for movement in all directions. Although the hip is considered a stable joint and is supported by many strong muscles, the large range of motion and mobility can make it susceptible to injury. Knowledge of basic hip anatomy is essential to understanding the different injuries that may occur in the hip and thigh. Due to the muscular attachments of the thigh muscles at the hip, many hip injuries can translate, or refer, pain into the thigh, low back, or both, thereby complicating the diagnostic process. This chapter provides a basic understanding of injuries common to the hip and thigh.

Anatomy Review

Bone structure:
Femur:
Greater trochanter, neck, head
Pelvis:
Ilium—iliac crest, anterior superior iliac spine (ASIS), posterior superior iliac spine (PSIS)
Pubis—attachment of adductors, occasional site for stress fracture
Ischium—ischial tuberosity, attachment of hamstrings

Ligamentous structure (see Figure 5.1):
Iliofemoral—Y ligament
Ischiofemoral
Pubofemoral
Inguinal ligament

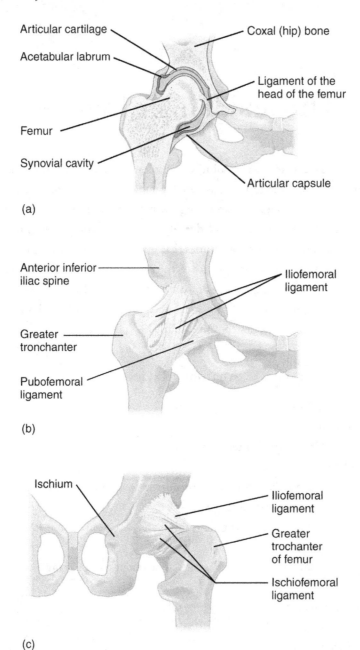

Figure 5.1 Bone and Ligament Anatomy of the Hip (a) Frontal section through the right hip joint; (b) Anterior view of right hip joint, capsule in place; and (c) Posterior view of right hip joint, capsule in place

Musculotendon structure (see Figures 5.2 to 5.5):

Extensors:

Gluteus maximus

Hamstrings

Flexors:

Iliopsoas

Pectineus

Rectus femoris—assists

Sartorius—assists

Tensor fascia latae—assists

Adductors:

Gracilis, pectineus

Adductor brevis, adductor longus, adductor magnus

Abductors:

Gluteus medius, gluteus minimus

Iliopsoas—assists

Sartorius

Tensor fascia latae

Internal rotators:

Adductors

Pectineus

External rotators:

Piriformis

Superior and inferior gemellus

Obturator internus and externus

Quadratus femoris

Other structures:

Trochanteric bursa

Acetabular labrum

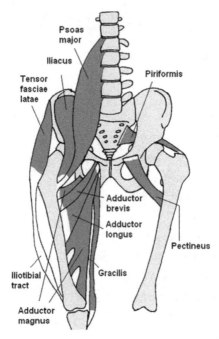

Figure 5.2 Muscle anatomy of the hip (deep)

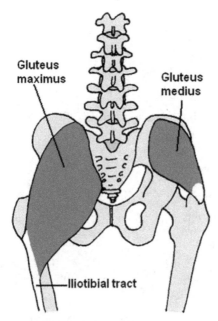

Figure 5.3 Gluteal muscles of the hip

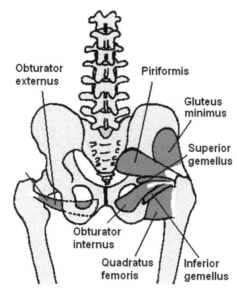

Figure 5.4 Muscle anatomy of the hip (rotators)

Injuries

Hamstring Strain

The hamstrings are a group of three muscles that run down the back of the leg and allow hip extension and knee flexion. All three muscles cross both the hip and knee joint. Hamstring strains can range from mild (partial tears) to severe (full ruptures) depending on the force and extent of the muscle damage. Hamstring strains often occur in soccer, basketball, track, and other sports that require explosive maneuvers such as rapid acceleration and deceleration. Strains are also common in underconditioned individuals who attempt explosive athletic maneuvers and are more common in those who have decreased flexibility, poor conditioning, muscle imbalance, and muscle fatigue, or any of these. More information regarding hamstring strains may be found in Table 5.1.

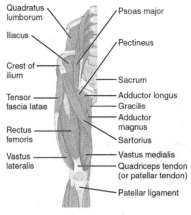

Superficial pelvic and thigh muscles
of right leg (anterior view)

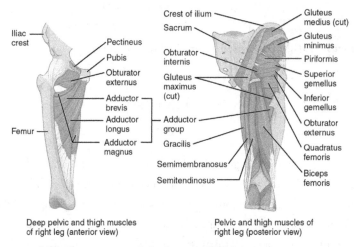

Deep pelvic and thigh muscles
of right leg (anterior view)

Pelvic and thigh muscles of
right leg (posterior view)

Figure 5.5 Muscle anatomy of the hip and thigh

Table 5.1 Hamstring strain

Mechanism of injury	Rapid overstretching of a muscle, sprinting, rapid deceleration
Signs and symptoms	Pain over the location of the strain, soreness, limping, swelling, discoloration, feeling of a pop, muscle weakness, possibly a divot if a rupture occurred
Treatment plan	Ice, compression, range-of-motion exercises, strengthening
Prevention strategies	Stretching, yoga, proper warm-up prior to activity

Quadriceps Strain

The quadriceps are a group of four muscles that cross both the hip and knee and are the primary muscles used to straighten the knee and are especially important for high speed running. Quadriceps strains can occur in any one or all of the four muscles. This injury can be sustained by athletes, as well as nonathletes, who overexert or attempt to produce more force than they are capable. Quadriceps strains are also attributed to poor flexibility, poor conditioning, muscle imbalances, muscle fatigue or any of these. Complications, such as myositis ossificans, can occur if return to activity occurs too soon after a severe muscle strain, and athletes with a quadriceps strain should be monitored for the development of calcification within the belly of the injured muscle. Information regarding quadriceps strains may be found in Table 5.2.

Table 5.2 **Quadriceps strain**

Mechanism of injury	Running, jumping, rapid overstretching
Signs and symptoms	Pain at the location of the strain, muscle weakness, feeling a pop, feeling a divot in severe strains
Treatment plan	Ice, compression, rest, cautious return to activity, range-of-motion exercises, strengthening exercises, watching for myositis ossificans development
Prevention strategies	Stretching, yoga, proper warm-up prior to activity

Femur Fracture

The femur is the longest bone in the body. A fracture to the femur is almost always caused by a direct blow and, typically, is the result of car accidents or a forceful collision with another object. Femur fractures can also occur as a result of falling, generally in elderly individuals with brittle bones. Fractures are named by the way they break, by the pattern of the break, or by the location of the break, but any femur fracture is considered a medical emergency as there is potential for irreversible arterial and nerve damage. It is essential to contact emergency medical services (EMS) immediately if a femoral fracture is suspected. Further management of this condition is shown in Table 5.3.

Table 5.3 Femur fracture

Mechanism of injury	Direct blow, car accident, direct blow with twisting, falling from a height, gunshot, severe osteoporosis
Signs and symptoms	Deformity, severe pain, shock, swelling, false joint, short leg, inability to move or bear weight
Treatment plan	Traction splint, surgery likely
Prevention strategies	Good bone health, none

Femoral Neck Stress Fracture

A femoral neck stress fracture often occurs with chronic impact stresses, such as high-mileage running. The "neck" of the femur is located between the ball and the shaft of the bone and is considered the weakest part of the femur. Fractures to the neck can be classified as displaced or nondisplaced. Nondisplaced stress fractures can either occur to the superior aspect of the neck (tension) or the inferior aspect of the neck (compression). Similar to stress fractures elsewhere in the body, a fracture of the femoral neck may not appear as on x-ray for up to three weeks post injury, once remodeling begins to take place. Considerations for management of this condition may be found in Table 5.4.

Table 5.4 Femoral neck stress fracture

Mechanism of injury	High-mileage running (distance or soccer); rapid increases in volume, intensity, or both, of running or other high-impact activity; osteoporosis
Signs and symptoms	Vague hip pain that cannot be palpated; deep ache, throbbing pain, or both; may feel worse with exercise and better when nonweight bearing
Treatment plan	Rest, nonweight-bearing activities, hip strengthening
Prevention strategies	Maintain good bone health, training and running on softer surfaces, cross-training such as cycling and aqua jogging

Trochanteric Bursitis

Trochanteric bursitis is the inflammation of the trochanteric bursa in the hip. Bursae are fluid-filled sacs that are located all over the body, especially in joint areas between bony prominences and tendons or other soft tissues. Bursae serve a protective role, providing cushion and preventing friction. The trochanteric bursa lies slightly behind the trochanter of the femur on the lateral side of the hip. Bursitis is generally considered an overuse injury and is common in sports such as volleyball and basketball where repetitive running and jumping occur. It is seen more commonly in females. Further information can be found in Table 5.5.

Table 5.5 Trochanteric bursitis

Mechanism of injury	Running, prolonged walking, excessive jumping, repetitive squatting
Signs and symptoms	Pain over the bursa and possibly down the thigh, swelling of the bursa, crepitus when moving the leg, pain when lying on the affected side at night, feeling stiff after sitting for long periods of time
Treatment plan	Ice, rest, heat, stretching, anti-inflammatory medications, activities that are pain-free, steroid injections
Prevention strategies	Cross-training, varying training surfaces, increase flexibility, increase strength, using proper shoes, maintaining healthy weight

Hip Dislocation: Posterior or Anterior

Hip dislocations are very painful and immediately debilitating. A dislocation of the hip occurs when the head of the femur is forced out of the socket of the joint. The hip typically dislocates in the posterior direction and rarely occurs anteriorly. When the hip dislocates, the surrounding skeletal structures also become misaligned and damage to soft tissue structures (muscles, cartilage, and ligaments) is common. Due to the possibility of damage to the arterial and nervous structures surrounding the hip, any hip dislocation is considered a medical emergency. It is extremely important to treat for shock and splint the leg in the position found. Never try to reduce a dislocated hip. Further information regarding this injury is shown in Table 5.6.

Table 5.6 Hip dislocation: posterior or anterior

Mechanism of injury	Axial load, high-impact force, car accident, falling from a height
Signs and symptoms	Severe pain, leg will appear shorter if posterior dislocation (internally rotated, adducted, and hip flexion), signs of shock (pallor, decreased blood pressure, and increased heart rate)
Treatment plan	Check femoral pulse, splint as is, activate EMS, treat for shock, hip reduction in the emergency room (ER), rehabilitation, regain strength
Prevention strategies	N/A

Iliac Crest and ASIS Contusion (Hip Pointer)

A hip pointer is a bruise to the iliac crest and surrounding soft tissue of the pelvis. It commonly occurs in athletes who play sports such as football, volleyball, and basketball. ASIS contusions are the result of a high-impact force striking the hip and, if forceful enough, can cause an avulsion fracture. This painful injury takes several weeks to heal but is generally managed conservatively with rest and ice until full mobility is restored. More information regarding this condition is shown in Table 5.7.

Table 5.7 Iliac crest and ASIS contusion

Mechanism of injury	Direct blow, landing on a hard surface with the hip
Signs and symptoms	Severe pain with movement of abdomen and legs; may be very limiting; discoloration over the pelvis; swelling; pain with laughing, coughing, or deep breathing
Treatment plan	Padding of the area, ice, rest, anti-inflammatory medications
Prevention strategies	Wear proper sporting equipment that fits well and do not alter protective sporting equipment in any way

Hernia: Inguinal or Femoral

Hernias generally result from a natural weakness in the abdominal muscles that is aggravated by a strain. An inguinal or femoral hernia is the result of the protrusion of the abdominal viscera through a portion of the abdominal muscles. Sometimes coughing, laughing, or "bearing down"

(Valsalva maneuver) will cause a hernia to become visible and painful. Hernias can be classified as either congenital, meaning present at birth, or acquired via activity. The majority of hernias that occur in males are inguinal hernias. Females more commonly experience femoral hernias. Hernias do not resolve or heal without surgery, and complications can occur if the bulging viscera get trapped by the abdominal muscles; if this happens, the portion of the bowel that is trapped can lose blood supply and die. This is referred to as strangulation. All femoral hernias are repaired immediately due to risk of strangulation, whereas, sometimes, inguinal hernias are not repaired as quickly. Management of these conditions is listed in Table 5.8.

Table 5.8 Hernia: inguinal or femoral

Mechanism of injury	Overstraining, heavy lifting, weak spot in the abdominal muscles, chronic coughing or sneezing, difficult bowel movement or constipation
Signs and symptoms	Previous history of injury, protrusion in groin area, protrusion can be increased by cough or bearing down, pain in the groin region, weakness or pulling sensation in groin area, sometimes there are no symptoms
Treatment plan	Surgery to avoid necrosis of the bowels or irritation from direct blow or falls
Prevention strategies	Proper lifting technique and abdominal strengthening, maintaining healthy weight, taking high-fiber diet to avoid constipation

Snapping Hip Syndrome

"Snapping hip" syndrome is a condition that presents with a snapping or popping sensation around the hip and can occur in three possible areas: internal, external, and within the intra-articular acetabular labrum. Internal "snapping hip" occurs when the iliopsoas tendon slips over the bony protrusions of the pelvis or when the iliofemoral ligament rides over the femoral head and results in a snapping sound that occurs at approximately 45° of flexion, when moving the hip from flexion to extension. This generally results from muscle tightness in the hip flexors.

The second type of "hip snapping" is external in location and occurs where the Iiliotibial band (IT band) or gluteus medius tendon becomes tight and "snaps" over the greater trochanter. External snapping can be felt on the outside of the hip during flexion and extension, and especially while the hip is internally rotated.

The third type of "snapping hip" syndrome is due to an intra-articular acetabular labral tear. In this case, the "snapping" sensation occurs deep within the joint when an axial load or pivoting movement occurs. An intra-articular tear will elicit a sharp pain in the groin and anterior thigh with this movement. This condition may require surgical intervention. Further explanation of these conditions are listed in Table 5.9.

Table 5.9 Snapping hip syndrome

Mechanism of injury	Tight hip muscles or IT band, chronic overuse of the hip joint (dancers). Axial load and pivot for intra-articular tears
Signs and symptoms	Snapping or popping in one of three locations (internal, external, or labrum); mild pain when internal, external, or both, snapping occurs; sharp pain if the labrum is torn
Treatment plan	Determine cause and location of the snapping, internal and external snapping responds positively to stretching of tight hip muscles and IT band, possible surgery if a labral tear is present
Prevention strategies	Maintain proper hip flexibility, cross-train, change training surfaces

Femoral Acetabular Impingement

Femoral acetabular impingement (FAI) occurs when the femoral head rubs abnormally on the acetabulum and is usually caused by an abnormal shape of the femoral head, the acetabulum, or both. Because the femoral head does not perfectly glide in the joint, repeated motion can eventually cause damage such as cartilage tears and early arthritis. There are three possible types of FAI: Cam deformity, Pincer deformity, or a combination of both, which are based on the location of the bone deformity. A Cam deformity means that there is excess bone on the femoral head and neck region that grinds on the labrum with any hip motion. A Pincer deformity is the result of excess bone on the rim of the acetabulum. The third possibility is a combination of both bone deformities on the femoral head and acetabulum. The result of either of the bone abnormalities is excessive wear and tear on the cartilage of the hip, which further causes tears of the labrum. Many people may have these deformities present in their hip but are unaware until symptoms appear. If conservative treatment fails, surgery will be needed to trim the bone deformity and clean up the damaged cartilage. Table 5.10 further describes the details of this condition.

Table 5.10 Femoral acetabular impingement

Mechanism of injury	Malformation of the hip bones during development, presents earlier in life of people who are more active, such as athletes
Signs and symptoms	Pain in the groin, can be sharp or stabbing pain with rotation, pivoting, or squatting, decreased range-of-motion, inability to perform activities of daily living without pain, limp
Treatment plan	Conservative (ROM, pain control, decrease aggravating activity), often surgical intervention is required
Prevention strategies	N/A

Hip Labral Tear

The labrum is a ring of cartilage that lines the acetabulum of the pelvis and forms the "socket" portion of the ball and socket joint of the hip. The cartilage ring acts to suction the head of the femur into the joint. Tears to this ring of cartilage are more common among dancers and gymnasts, as well as traditional team sport athletes. The mechanism of injury is usually an axial load and generally surgery is required to repair this poorly vascularized area. Diagnosis is difficult thus requires additional imaging. The condition is further described in Table 5.11.

Table 5.11 Hip labral tear

Mechanism of injury	Axial load while weight bearing (trauma), chronic hip stress, FAI (see earlier discussion), unknown
Signs and symptoms	Snapping or catching sensations, locking sensation, pain with hip rotation, pain deep in the groin region
Treatment plan	Surgery to repair or remove the torn portion of the labrum
Prevention strategies	N/A

Bibliography

"AAOS—OrthoInfo." n.d. www.orthoinfo.aaos.org/ (accessed January 7, 2016).

Bahr, R., and L. Engebretsen. 2009. *Sports Injury Prevention*. Chichester, UK: Wiley-Blackwell.

"Diseases and Conditions." n.d. www.mayoclinic.org/diseases-conditions (accessed January 7, 2016).

Guanche, C.A. 2010. *Hip & Pelvis Injuries in Sports Medicine*. Philadelphia, PA: Wolters Kluwer Health/Lippincott Williams & Wilkins.

CHAPTER 6

Lumbar Spine Injuries

Low back injuries are common among active as well as sedentary populations and is the most common site for back pain and injuries, which can include: strains, sprains, disc injuries, and vertebral fractures. Often these injuries are the result of poor core strength and tight musculature surrounding the hip and low back. The majority of people will, at some point, experience low back pain, an injury, or both, which will result in discomfort, inability to participate in sport, and diminished ability to perform activities of daily living. In order to prevent low back injury, it is essential to understand the anatomy of the spine, recognize the movements and postures associated with injury, and learn proper lifting techniques. This chapter describes the various conditions associated with the lower back and provides recommendations for injury prevention and treatment.

Anatomy Review

Bone structure (see Figure 6.1):
   Cervical vertebrae (7)
   Thoracic vertebrae (12)
   Lumbar vertebrae (5)
   Sacrum (five fused bones make up one sacrum)
   Coccyx (three to five fused bones make up one coccyx)
   Pelvis:
      Ilium—(iliac crest, anterior superior iliac spine [ASIS], posterior superior iliac spine [PSIS])
      Pubis (attachment of adductors, occasional site for stress fracture)
      Ischium with ischial tuberosity (attachment of hamstrings)

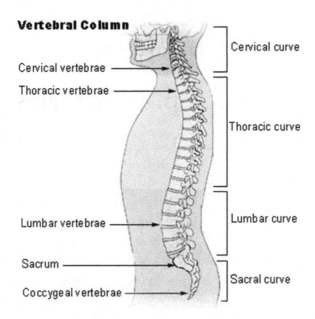

Figure 6.1 Vertebral column

Landmarks on the vertebrae (see Figure 6.2):
    Body
    Pedicles
    Lamina
    Transverse process
    Spinous process
    Vertebral foramen (spinal canal)
    Intervertebral foramen
    Superior articular process (facets or articular surfaces)
    Inferior articular process (facets or articular surfaces)

Musculotendon structure:
    Erector spinae—(iliocostalis, longissimus, spinalis)
    Transversospinalis—(semispinalis, multifidus)
    Quadratus lumborum

Serratus posterior inferior—(respiratory muscles—beneath latissimus dorsi)

Rectus abdominus

External obliques

Internal obliques

Transverse abdominus—(deepest, compresses abdominal contents)

Other structures:

Intervertebral discs (see Figure 6.3)

Sciatic nerve (see Figure 6.4)

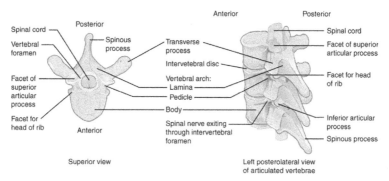

Figure 6.2 *Vertebrae anatomy*

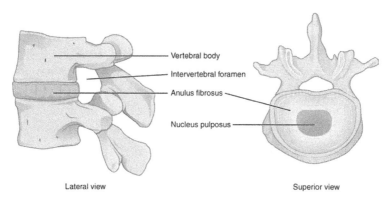

Figure 6.3 *Vertebral disc anatomy*

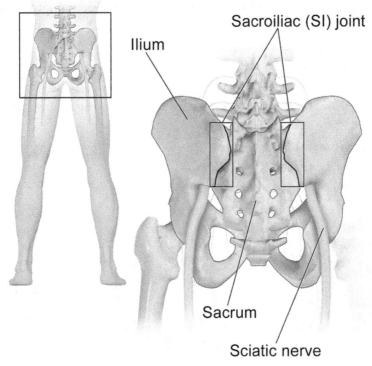

Figure 6.4 Sciatic nerve

Injuries

Disc Pathology

Disc pathology encompasses a variety of possible injuries to discs that serve to separate and cushion the vertebrae. These injuries are often termed bulging discs, herniated discs, or slipped discs based on findings revealed on diagnostic imaging. Injuries to the disc become more likely with age because of the loss of interdisc water content. The majority of disc injuries occur in between L4–L5 or L5–S1.

The synonymous terms bulging disc, disc herniation, and disc slippage all involve the nucleus of the disc being pushing out onto the outer rings of the annulus; eventually, the disc can push onto peripheral nerves and beyond. Herniation of the disc can range from mild to severe depending on the degree of disc displacement. Typically, people with disc injuries who are also overweight have increased pain due to compressive

Table 6.1 Disc pathology

Mechanism of injury	Trunk flexion with rotation, repetitive movement, improper lifting techniques, overweight, axial load
Signs and symptoms	General low back pain, low back pain radiating below the knee, decreased sensation in specific areas of the lower extremities, pain with straight leg raise at 30°–45°, decreased reflexes in area, signs and symptoms reproduced with trunk flexion, weak leg muscles in associated area
Treatment plan	Rest, ice, bracing, anti-inflammatory medications, back extension exercises, general aerobic conditioning, decrease weight, core strengthening
Prevention strategies	Maintain healthy weight, use proper lifting techniques, maintain core strength

forces being placed on the disk by excess weight. Additional description and treatment plan for this condition this condition can be found in Table 6.1.

Spondylolysis or Spondylolisthesis

Spondylolysis or spondylolisthesis are both related to degeneration and stress fracture of the pars interarticularis in the vertebral body. These conditions are often generally referred to as "spondys," but there are apparent differences between the two terms. If a person has a spondylolysis, there is stress fracture but without slippage of the vertebral body. In a spondylolisthesis, there is a fracture in addition to anterior slippage of the vertebral body. The amount of slippage can be graded as first, second, or third degree, with third degree being the most severe and having greater potential for neurological pathology. In the athletic population, spondys are more commonly seen in athletes who participate in gymnastics or other sports that require excessive back extension (such as football lineman). More information regarding this condition is presented in Table 6.2.

Facet Joint Sprain

Facet joints are found along the spinal column on each side of the vertebrae. They serve as attachment points for numerous ligaments and

Table 6.2 Spondylolysis or spondylolisthesis

Mechanism of injury	Degeneration over time, overuse, repeated back extension or hyperextension activities
Signs and symptoms	Pain with back extension, general back pain, general stiffness Spondylolisthesis: lower vertebra may appear to protrude posteriorly but actually affected vertebra has moved anteriorly, palpate step off deformity (sinking in of vertebrae)
Treatment plan	Low back and core strengthening exercises, anti-inflammatory medications, rehab with progression as tolerated for chronic pain, general rehab to decrease pain and stiffness
Prevention strategies	Avoid aggravating postures and correct biomechanical abnormalities, maintain core strength and healthy weight

Table 6.3 Facet sprain

Mechanism of injury	Excessive bending, lifting, twisting, overuse, poor posture
Signs and symptoms	Sudden or gradual onset of pain, sharp pain when the facet joint is stressed, may have no pain when the facet joint is not stressed, muscle spasm, pain radiating to lateral and anterior thigh, pain with rotation and extension, pain is specific to a location near the spine
Treatment plan	Treat the symptoms with ice, heat, stretching, low back strengthening, postural evaluation, core strengthening
Prevention strategies	Maintain healthy weight, use proper lifting techniques, maintain muscle strength and flexibility

muscles, allowing for stability and motion of the spine. A sprain to the facet joint occurs in any of the connective tissue surrounding the joint and is a painful injury that presents similar to a strain or fracture but rarely does it involve the spinal nerves. There will be no palpable deformity but the joint will be painful to the touch and the athlete will not want to fully extend the spine. Pain may be relieved by taking pressure off the facet by means of stretching and traction. Facet sprains are commonly seen in football players, gymnasts, and dancers. Management of this condition is presented in Table 6.3.

Piriformis Syndrome and Sciatica

Overuse of the piriformis muscle, which is responsible for externally rotating and abducting the thigh, is commonly seen in individuals who

Table 6.4 Piriformis syndrome and sciatica

Mechanism of injury	Overuse, excessive running, trauma to the gluteal muscles (falling on your buttocks), tight piriformis muscle, sitting for prolonged times (truck drivers, motor bikers, cyclists)
Signs and symptoms	Pain in the gluteals, pain with resisted external rotation, tight internal rotation, intolerance to sitting, muscle weakness If the sciatic nerve is compressed, numbness, tingling, and burning occurs in the glutes and radiates down the back of the leg
Treatment plan	Stretch the piriformis, soft tissue massage, alter activity, anti-inflammatory medications
Prevention strategies	Practice proper lifting techniques; increase flexibility and strength in the hamstrings, glutes, and piriformis

perform activities that involve running, skating, cross-country skiing, cycling, or other activities that require hip stability. To test for the condition, it is essential to isolate the muscle. Often additional stabilizing muscles of the hip can also be affected with piriformis syndrome.

Piriformis syndrome is usually accompanied by low back pain. Sciatica or "lumbosacral radicular syndrome" occurs when the sciatic nerve is compressed (commonly by the piriformis muscle) and therefore causes radiating pain into the buttocks and down the back of the leg. This can also be the result of muscular tightness or nerve entrapment due to a lumbar spine injury. The term sciatica is broad by nature, and it is essential to find the cause of the nerve compression in order to treat the condition. Further description and management of these conditions are presented in Table 6.4.

Muscle Strain of the Low Back

A muscle strain in the low back is usually diagnosed after everything else has been ruled out or when the signs and symptoms do not warrant further assessment (e.g., x-rays, magnetic resonance imaging, bone scan). Low back strains occur when the muscles of the low back are rapidly overstretched, and pain typically follows the length of the muscle without radiating down the legs. Generally speaking, individuals who experience a muscle strain in the low back can associate the initiation of symptoms with a specific event that included some type of eccentric

Table 6.5 Muscle strain

Mechanism of injury	Overstretching, lifting heavy object, lifting while twisting, sudden movements, fall
Signs and symptoms	Painful to touch, stiffness, pain may be intense with movement, muscle spasm, inability to move
Treatment plan	Stretch, ice, electrical stimulation, ultrasound, anti-inflammatory medications, muscle relaxers
Prevention strategies	Maintain healthy weight, use proper lifting techniques, maintain core strength

loading of the muscles. There is generally no specific mechanism of injury, and symptoms will decrease with rest over a short period of time but are often recurring. Further description of this injury can be found in Table 6.5.

Basic Strengthening Exercises for the Low Back and Core

The following exercises may be used for the prevention of, or rehabilitation from, a back injury and are designed to facilitate improvements in low back range of motion, neuromuscular control, and strength.

A. *Maintaining and reestablishing range of motion*:
   a. Maintaining joint flexibility is an important aspect in the prevention of injuries. After a low back injury, regaining movement is important to progress the rehabilitation process and return to normal activities.
   b. Stretches should be held for 20 to 30 seconds and be repeated bilaterally two to three times daily.
      i.   Hamstrings
      ii.   Hip flexors
      iii. Glutes
      iv.   Calves
      v.   IT band
      vi.   Piriformis
      vii. Prayer stretch

B. *Maintaining or reestablishing core strength*:
   a. Exercises options include:
      i.   Pelvic tilts
      ii. Bridging
      iii. Bird dogs
      iv. Supermans
      v.   Crunches: forward, diagonal
      vi. Extension
      vii. Planks

C. *Maintaining and reestablishing back, hip, and leg strength*:
   a. Increasing the strength of the muscles around the low back will help provide support to the ligaments and joint and can help prevent future injury
   b. A basic rehabilitation protocol generally includes:
      i.   Three sets of 10 repetitions of each exercise with 30 to 90 seconds between each set
      ii. Three times per week with at least 48 hours between sessions
      iii. Exercises can be completed using no weight initially and then progressing to light ankle weights or weight machines
   c. Muscles to be targeted include:
      i.   Glutes (hip extension, with internal rotation and external rotation)
      ii. Hamstrings (leg curl)
      iii. Gastrocnemius and soleus complex (toe raises)
      iv. Anterior tibialis (ankle dorsiflexion)
      v.   Rectus abdominus and transverse abdominus (crunches)
      vi. Erector spinae (back extension)
      vii. Obliques (crunch with rotation)

D. *Maintaining and reestablishing balance*:
   Exercises are listed from easiest (a) to most challenging (c). Each of the following balance exercises should initially be performed for 30 seconds and progressively increase in duration until the posture can easily be maintained for one minute. Once mastery of the easy

skills has been achieved, progression to a more difficult balance skill can be initiated. Exercises should be performed at least three times each week and preferably every day.

1. Progressive sequence of balance exercises:
    a. One-legged stance on a flat surface
    b. One-legged stance on a flat surface with eyes closed
    c. One-legged stance on an uneven surface (pillow, mini trampoline, etc.)

Bibliography

"AAOS—OrthoInfo." n.d. www.orthoinfo.aaos.org/ (accessed January 7, 2016).

"Diseases and Conditions." n.d. www.mayoclinic.org/diseases-conditions (accessed January 7, 2016).

Houglum, P.A. 2010. *Therapeutic Exercise for Musculoskeletal Injuries*. Champaign, IL: Human Kinetics.

Park, J.Y. 2015. *Sports Injuries to the Shoulder and Elbow*. Berlin: Springer.

Wilk, K.E., M.M. Reinold, and J.R. Andrews. 2009. *The Athlete's Shoulder*. Philadelphia, PA: Churchill Livingstone/Elsevier. www.clinicalkey.com/dura/browse/bookChapter/3-s2.0-B9780443067013X50014

PART II
Upper Extremity

CHAPTER 7

Shoulder Injuries

The shoulder is a ball-and-socket joint that is among the most dynamic and complex joints in the body. The shoulder is inherently unstable due to the structure of the joint, but is supported by a number of muscles and a ligamentous capsule. Any injury to the musculature or capsule can cause joint instability. Shoulder injuries are very common in sports and activities that require repetitive, overhead motions and are most commonly seen in athletes who participate in baseball, softball, tennis, swimming, and lifting weights. A review of the shoulder anatomy is shown in Figures 7.1 to 7.5 and will facilitate assessment and recognition of injury to specific regions in this complex joint structure.

Anatomy Review

Bone structure (see Figure 7.1):
Sternum
Humerus
    Head, greater and lesser tubercles, bicipital groove
Scapula
    Spine, superior and inferior angles, medial and lateral borders, acromion and coracoid processes, fossas
Clavicle

Joints:
Sternoclavicular joint (SC)
Acromioclavicular joint (AC)
Glenohumeral joint (GH)
Scapulothoracic joint (ST)

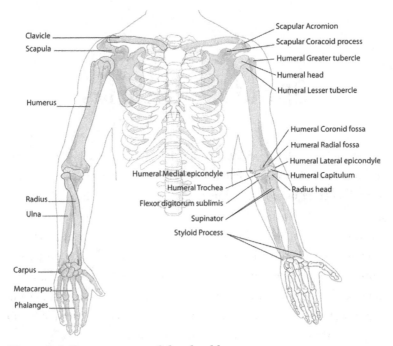

Clavicle
Scapula
Humerus
Radius
Ulna
Carpus
Metacarpus
Phalanges

Scapular Acromion
Scapular Coracoid process
Humeral Greater tubercle
Humeral head
Humeral Lesser tubercle
Humeral Coronid fossa
Humeral Radial fossa
Humeral Lateral epicondyle
Humeral Capitulum
Radius head

Humeral Medial epicondyle
Humeral Trochea
Flexor digitorum sublimis
Supinator
Styloid Process

Figure 7.1 Bone anatomy of the shoulder

Musculotendon structure (see Figure 7.2):

Biceps

Triceps

Deltoids

     Anterior, middle, posterior

Latissimus dorsi

Trapezius

     Upper, middle, lower

Rhomboids

     Major and minor

Serratus anterior

Levator scapulae

Pectoralis major and minor

Rotator cuff muscles

     1. Supraspinatus

     2. Infraspinatus

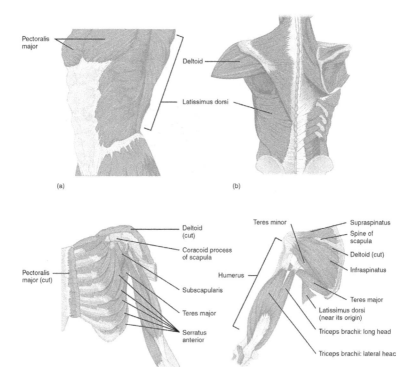

Figure 7.2 Muscle anatomy of the shoulder and trunk: (a) pectoralis major and latissimus dorsi (left anterior view); (b) left deltoid left latissimus dorsi (posterior view); (c) deep muscles of the left shoulder (anterior lateral view); and (d) deep muscles of the left shoulder (posterior view)

3. Teres minor
4. Subscapularis

Other structure:

Glenoid labrum (see Figure 7.3)

Bursa (see Figure 7.4):

1. Subacromial-subdeltoid
2. Subscapular
3. Subcoracoid
4. Coracoclavicular

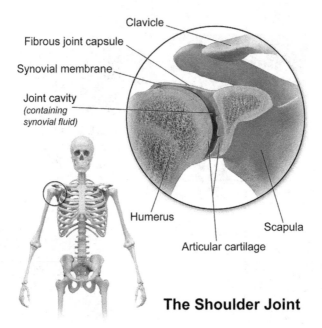

Clavicle

Fibrous joint capsule

Synovial membrane

Joint cavity
(containing
synovial fluid)

Humerus

Scapula

Articular cartilage

The Shoulder Joint

Figure 7.3 Glenohumeral joint and labrum anatomy

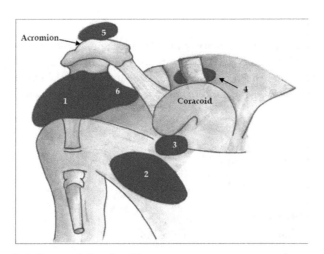

Acromion

Coracoid

Figure 7.4 Bursa of the shoulder

5. Supra-acromial

6. Medial extension of subacromial-subdeltoid bursa

Brachial plexus (see Figure 7.5)

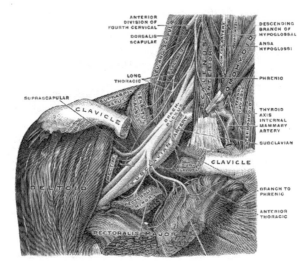

Figure 7.5 Brachial plexus

Injuries

SC Joint Sprain

SC joint sprains occur where the medial clavicle and the sternum join together. Severity of SC injury is graded from first to third degree. Most commonly, a first or second degree sprain occurs to the anterior, posterior, or superior portions of the ligament. If enough force is applied to the SC joint, a third degree sprain could occur, which results in a separation of the joint. If the clavicle is displaced posteriorly, it will present with dizziness and difficulty breathing, and is considered a medical emergency. SC joint sprains generally result from falling on an outstretched hand, direct blow to the lateral aspect of the shoulder, or in some instances by traction applied to the arm; however, traction injuries are considered rare. More information regarding this condition can be found in Table 7.1.

AC Joint Sprain

AC joint sprains occur quite commonly in the shoulder. Severity of joint separation is graded from first to third degree and the injury can happen acutely or over time. AC joint sprains present with pain on top of the

Table 7.1 SC joint sprain

Signs and symptoms	Pain during joint motion, protraction and retraction reproduce pain First degree sprains will have no deformity, point tenderness, slight pain with rotation Second degree sprains will have some displacement, point tenderness with swelling, movement is painful, especially with arm rotation Third degree sprains will have complete displacement and arm movement will cause severe pain
Treatment	Rest and limit motion to the shoulder and arm by wearing a sling, which sometimes relieves pain in the joint
Prevention strategies	N/A

shoulder and commonly the patient will hold their arm close to their body to support the sprain. If severe enough, the sprain can cause a "step deformity" at the joint, wherein the articulation between the acromion and clavicle will look like a stair step. Sometimes the deformity of a distal clavicle fracture may look like an AC joint sprain but can be distinguished by special tests performed by a trained medical professional. AC sprains are common in hockey players when they get boarded into the glass or in other contact sports where an athlete falls on the outer tip of the shoulder. The most common mechanism for an AC sprain is a force that causes the acromion to be driven away from clavicle via a direct blow from the top or the outside of the shoulder. See Table 7.2 for management of this injury.

GH Instability

The GH joint is the ball-and-socket joint of the shoulder. It is surrounded by a ligamentous capsule that provides joint stability throughout joint motion. The GH joint capsule can incur instability to the anterior, posterior, or inferior aspect, or in any combination of these directions. However, the majority occurs anteriorly, as there is less protection to the joint in this direction and the anterior capsule is commonly stressed in overhead activities. It is essential to know the portion of the capsule that is unstable in order to treat the condition. After the initial GH injury, the joint becomes inherently weak and more susceptible to future injuries, especially subluxation or dislocation or both. GH instability usually

Table 7.2 AC joint sprain

Signs and symptoms	Point tenderness over the AC joint, swelling, pain with arm movement First degree sprains: AC ligament injured only, no laxity, pain with palpation and horizontal adduction Second degree sprains: AC ligament and CC lgament are involved, laxity, pain with palpation and horizontal adduction, slight step deformity Third degree sprain: AC ligament and CC lgament are torn completely, step deformity, laxity, decreased function, weakness
Treatment plan	Avoid aggravating activity and decrease shoulder movement with a sling. In some instances, additional padding will be necessary to prevent further injury in contact sports. Strengthening the musculature around the shoulder will allow for increased stability, but the ligaments will remain unstable without surgical intervention
Prevention strategies	Coaching for appropriate tackling techniques and falling correctly, strengthening of the shoulder muscles

Table 7.3 GH instability

Signs and symptoms	Pain or clicking in the GH, decreased or excessive translation of the humeral head in the direction of the weakness, decreased range of motion, feelings of instability in the shoulder joint
Treatment plan	Strengthening and scapular stabilization, functional exercises and multidirectional activity, avoid overhead movement until joint is stable
Prevention strategies	Rotator cuff strengthening and scapular stabilization Maintaining good posture and strengthening muscles surrounding the shoulder complex

results from poor mechanics or weak musculature in the shoulder coupled with repetitive overhead activity (swimming and throwing) or an outside force such as a direct blow or falling on an outstretched arm. In some cases, congenital weakness can cause the GH joint to be unstable. More information regarding instability can be found in Table 7.3.

Shoulder Subluxation or Dislocation (GH)

As mentioned previously, a shoulder subluxation or dislocation is often the result of GH instability. Because the shoulder joint is dynamic and inherently unstable, this injury is one of the most common orthopedic injuries. Subluxation refers to a joint that has moved out of place and returns to its original position without external force placed upon it or reduction. Dislocation refers to a joint that has moved out of place and stays out of place. In the event of a dislocation, reduction must be performed by a medical professional. Subluxations and dislocations can also be associated with trauma of some sort, such as a direct blow or arm tackling in football or rugby. Table 7.4 shows additional information regarding this condition.

Table 7.4 Shoulder subluxation or dislocation

Signs and symptoms	Pain, deformity evident in the shoulder that usually results in a flattened deltoid, inability to move the arm
Treatment plan	Reduction of dislocation, anti-inflammatory medication, strengthening of the shoulder musculature, gradual return to activity; bracing may be necessary to help provide increased stability Recurrent dislocations will often lead to surgical intervention to tighten the affected ligaments
Prevention strategies	Rotator cuff strengthening and scapular stabilization. Maintaining good posture and strengthening muscles surrounding the shoulder complex

Rotator Cuff Tendinopathy

The rotator cuff provides stability in the shoulder for rotational movement. The "cuff" itself consists of four muscles: the supraspinatus, infraspinatus, teres minor, and subscapularis. If any of the four muscles is compromised, the athlete will experience weakness and inability to complete rotational movements, such as throwing. The rotator cuff is often injured as a result of overuse, and this injury is more common in adults than in teens or children. In extreme cases, the rotator cuff can be surgically repaired but a conservative approach is often successful. Recognition and treatment information for this condition can be found in Table 7.5.

Table 7.5 Rotator cuff tendinopathy

Signs and symptoms	Point tenderness over the affected muscle with inability to use the muscle when isolated, limited range of motion Sometimes the patient will feel popping with rotational movement in the shoulder
Treatment plan	Decrease pain, anti-inflammatory medications Begin isolated rotator cuff exercises with elastic tubing in flexion, extension, internal rotation, and external rotation, work back into dynamic activities, such as throwing, swimming
Prevention strategies	Correct throwing mechanics and strengthening

Impingement and Bursitis

An impingement occurs when there is a decrease in the amount of space through which the rotator cuff muscles and tendon can pass. Initial stages result in rotator cuff inflammation, which decreases the space and thus adds to the irritation of the rotator cuff muscles and underlying bursae. The mechanism for this injury generally changes with age. In patients under 35 years old, impingement and bursitis are commonly associated with overhead sports or shoulder instability. In patients over 35 years old, degeneration of joint structures is often the primary cause for impingement or bursitis. Either way, as the joint space is minimized and underlying structures are trapped, the patient will experience an inability to move the joint through a full range of motion and will experience additional symptoms. This condition is outlined further in Table 7.6.

Table 7.6 Impingement and bursitis

Signs and symptoms	Pain with overhead activities, weakness
Treatment plan	Decrease inflammation, anti-inflammatory medication, gradual return to range of motion, strengthen rotator cuff muscles below the shoulder level first, then move toward overhead activity
Prevention strategies	Maintain rotator cuff strength and increase flexibility in the shoulder complex

Clavicle Fracture

Clavicle fractures result from falls or accidents and are more common in children than in adults. The most common fracture site occurs where the bone changes direction at the middle third of the structure. This injury is generally sustained from a direct blow or a fall on an outstretched arm. The clavicle will often be displaced with this type of injury and may require surgical intervention and hardware to regain continuity in the joint. Often the hardware will cause irritation after the bone heals and a second surgery will be required to remove screws or plates that were initially placed to aid healing. Table 7.7 describes this condition further and offers treatment suggestions.

Table 7.7 Clavicle fracture

Signs and symptoms	Deformity apparent at the fracture site, decreased arm strength, pain, swelling, bruising, pain with arm movement
Treatment plan	Sling, butterfly or figure 8 harness to pull shoulders back, rehabilitation, possible surgery to put in a plate in severe cases
Prevention strategies	Teach appropriate tackling and falling techniques

Burners or Stingers

A burner, or stinger, is the result of overstretching or compressing the nerves in the brachial plexus of the neck. This injury is common in tackling, especially in football defensive players and linebackers. Generally, a stinger results from traction or compression of the brachial plexus; this can happen if the neck is forced sideways or by a direct blow to Erb's point, which lies halfway between the neck and shoulder. This injury often results in temporary numbness, weakness, and tingling in the shoulder. Symptoms usually resolve within a few minutes but if the injury happens multiple times, resolution can take longer. It is essential to cease participation in activity while symptoms are present, as the athlete will not be able to protect the shoulder from injury if numbness or weakness is present. Table 7.8 gives further guidance for treating this injury.

Table 7.8 Burners or stingers

Signs and symptoms	Burning or tingling sensation around the neck, down the arm, or into the hand. Numbness or tingling surrounding the arm, but only affects one arm. This does not follow dermatomal pattern, and may cause muscle weakness or point tenderness over Erb's point
Treatment plan	Numbness or tingling usually resolves in 1 to 2 minutes without intervention; decreased strength and range of motion may linger Repeated or more severe nerve injury may result in permanent nerve damage
Prevention strategies	Neck roll padding or cowboy collar for football or sports involving shoulder pads

Shoulder Strengthening

By strengthening the shoulder musculature, many injuries can be prevented. The basic exercises used in shoulder strengthening involve internal rotation, external rotation, flexion, and extension. Each of the following exercises can be performed using either elastic tubing or light hand weights (no more than five pounds). Exercises can be performed daily and generally three sets of 10 repetitions for each exercise are adequate for prevention.

Internal Rotation

Starting position:

A. Stand tall with your shoulder blades squeezed together
B. Squeeze a towel between the elbow and ribs
C. Elbow should be bent to 90 degrees
D. Start with the arm rotated away from the trunk

Movement:

A. Rotate the shoulder inward bringing the arm toward the belly button
B. Slowly rotate back to the starting position
C. Repeat the motion 10 times

External Rotation

Starting position:

A. Stand tall with shoulder blades squeezed together
B. Squeeze a towel between the elbow and ribs
C. Elbow bent to 90 degrees
D. Start with arm rotated in, close to your trunk

Movement:

A. Rotate the shoulder outward, away from the belly button
B. Slowly rotate back to the starting position
C. Repeat the motion 10 times

Flexion (see Figure 7.6a and b)

Starting position:

A. Stand tall with shoulder blades squeezed together
B. Elbow extended (straight)
C. Thumb at hip level

Movement:

A. Keeping the elbow extended, bring the arm forward from the hip to shoulder level
B. Slowly lower back to the starting position
C. Repeat the motion 10 times

Extension (See Figure 7.6a and b)

Starting position:

A. Stand tall with shoulder blades squeezed together
B. Elbow extended (straight)
C. Thumb at hip level

Movement:

A. Keeping the elbow extended, extend the arm back from the hip
B. Slowly return to the starting position
C. Repeat the motion 10 times

Abduction (see Figure 7.6e)

Starting position:

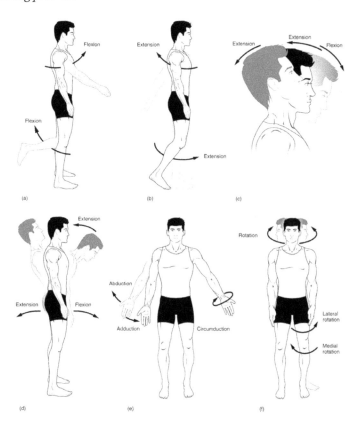

Figure 7.6 Anatomical motions of the shoulder: (a) and (b) angular movements: flexion and extension at the shoulder and knees; (c) angular movements: flexion extension of the neck; (d) angular movements: flexion and extension of the vertebral column; (e) angular movements: abduction, adduction, and circumduction of the upper limb at the shoulder; and (f) rotation of the head, neck, and lower limb

A. Stand tall with shoulder blades squeezed together

B. Elbow extended (straight)

C. Thumb at hip level

Movement:

A. Keeping the elbow extended, move the arm into abduction (away from the body) up to shoulder level

B. Slowly return to the starting position

C. Repeat the motion 10 times

Bibliography

"AAOS—OrthoInfo." n.d. www.orthoinfo.aaos.org/ (accessed January 7, 2016).

"Diseases and Conditions." n.d. www.mayoclinic.org/diseases-conditions (accessed January 7, 2016).

Houglum, P.A. 2010. *Therapeutic Exercise for Musculoskeletal Injuries*. Champaign, IL: Human Kinetics.

Park, J.Y. 2015. *Sports Injuries to the Shoulder and Elbow*. Berlin, Germany: Springer.

Wilk, K.E., M.M. Reinold, and J.R. Andrews. 2009. *The Athlete's Shoulder*. Philadelphia, PA: Churchill Livingstone/Elsevier. www.clinicalkey.com/dura/browse/bookChapter/3-s2.0-B9780443067013X50014

CHAPTER 8

Elbow Injuries

The elbow is actually a combination of three joints that are all encompassed by the same joint capsule; therefore, when a person has an injury to one of the joints, the whole elbow and all of its motions are affected. These injuries can range from minor to severe and are often due to overuse activities. Athletes who throw or play racquet sports are especially susceptible to elbow injuries. Often, the ligaments supporting the elbow are injured by valgus or varus force or hyperextension. Similar to other joints, if the stabilizing structures for the elbow are injured, the joint becomes more susceptible to further injury. This chapter describes the anatomy of the elbow joint and some of the more common injuries seen in this structure.

Anatomy Review

Bone structure (see Figure 8.1):
Humerus
Medial and lateral epicondyle, capitulum, trochlea, olecranon fossa
Radius
Head
Ulna
Olecranon process, coronoid process

Joints:
Ulnohumeral joint
Radiohumeral joint   All have continuous joint capsule
Radioulnar joint

Ligaments:
Radial collateral ligament
Ulnar collateral ligament (UCL)
Annular ligament

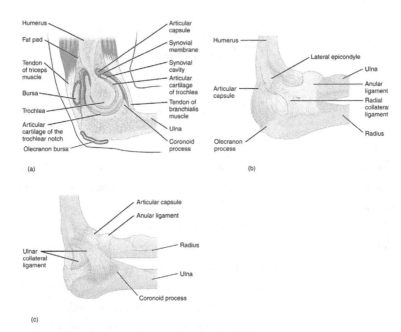

Figure 8.1 Elbow anatomy: (a) medial sagittal section through right elbow (lateral view); (b) lateral view of right elbow joint; and (c) medial view of right elbow joint

Musculotendon structure (see Figure 8.2):

> Biceps
> Triceps and anconeus
> Common wrist flexors
> Common wrist extensors
> Pronators
> Supinators

Other structure:

> Nerves (see Figure 8.3):
>> Musculocutaneous nerve
>> Radial nerve

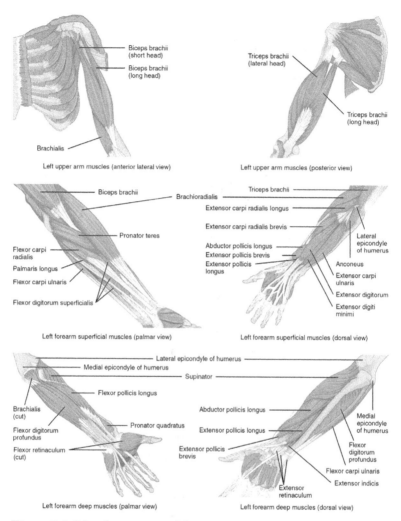

Figure 8.2 Muscle anatomy of the arm

Median nerve

Ulnar nerve

Bursa:

Olecranon

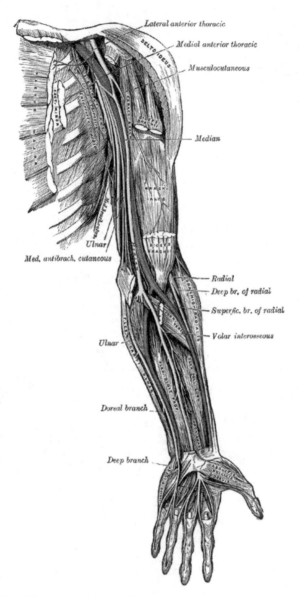

Figure 8.3 Nerve anatomy of the arm

Injuries

Medial Epicondylitis

Medial epicondylitis is a common injury seen in active populations and is often termed "golfer's elbow." This overuse injury involves the wrist flexors, and pain is localized over the medial epicondyle of the elbow. Pain is reproduced by activities such as swinging a golf club, pitching, and javelin throwing. Recognition and management of this condition are shown in Table 8.1.

Table 8.1 Medial epicondylitis

Signs and symptoms	Point tender at the medial epicondyle, weak wrist flexion, pain with passive wrist extension and overpressure, occasional swelling at the medial epicondyle
Treatment plan	Rest, stretch the wrist flexors, ultrasound for chronic inflammation or pain, anti-inflammatory medications, taping, or bracing
Prevention strategies	Stretching and strengthening wrist flexors

Lateral Epicondylitis

Lateral epicondylitis is another common elbow injury and is often termed "tennis elbow." This overuse injury involves the wrist extensors, and pain is localized over the lateral epicondyle of the elbow. Pain is reproduced by activities such as a backhand swing in tennis, wrist extension, excessive curveball pitching, power grips, or by impact forces such as operating a drill. Further information describing this injury is shown in Table 8.2.

Table 8.2 Lateral epicondylitis

Signs and symptoms	Point tender over the lateral epicondyle, weak wrist extension, pain with passive flexion overpressure, occasional swelling at the lateral epicondyle, decreased grip strength
Treatment plan	Rest, stretching the wrist extensors, ultrasound for chronic inflammation or pain, anti inflammatory medication, taping or bracing, two-handed backhand in tennis
Prevention strategies	Stretching and strengthening wrist extensors

Olecranon Bursitis

Olecranon bursitis involves inflammation of the olecranon bursa, which lies directly beneath the skin and on top of the olecranon process. Injury to this bursa will cause pain and immediate inflammation. This injury can be acute or as a result of overuse. Acute injury to the bursa can be a result of a direct blow to the tip of the elbow or from falling on the elbow. Chronic injury typically involves resting the elbow on a table or desk and is termed "student's elbow". On rare occasions, the bursa can become infected, which causes inflammation and presents with other signs of infection such as warmth, pain, and redness. Additional description of this condition is provided in Table 8.3.

Table 8.3 Olecranon bursitis

Signs and symptoms	Obvious swelling within the bursa over the olecranon, range of motion may be limited because of swelling, especially in flexion
Treatment plan	Pad, ice, compression, occasionally the bursitis will need to be drained by a medical professional using a hypodermic needle
Prevention strategies	N/A

Ulnar Nerve Palsy ("Funny Bone")

Ulnar nerve palsy is more commonly known as "hitting the funny bone." The mechanism of injury is a direct blow to the ulnar nerve, hitting the medial elbow, or landing on the elbow. Other mechanisms for nerve palsy include habitual resting of the elbows on a table or desk, excessive stretch placed on the ulnar nerve, or leading with the elbow when throwing or pitching. The symptoms of this condition generally dissipate within minutes. Further information is listed in Table 8.4.

Table 8.4 Ulnar nerve palsy

Signs and symptoms	Typically transitory tingling that may radiate into the hand (pinky side), lasting numbness or tingling is a concern
Treatment plan	Ice, rest, stretch flexor muscles, limit elbow extension. Pad the elbow for protection if necessary for sport
Prevention strategies	Wearing elbow pads for activities

Ulnar Nerve Entrapment (Cubital Tunnel Syndrome)

The ulnar nerve, as it runs through the elbow, can become entrapped, compressed, and irritated. Compression of the nerve can cause pain and numbness and is considered an overuse injury. This condition is especially common in those who play racket sports and those who throw by leading with the elbow. If a person has an ulnar nerve entrapment, symptoms will get progressively worse and may require surgical intervention. The signs, symptoms, and treatment for this condition are listed in Table 8.5.

Table 8.5 Ulnar nerve entrapment

Signs and symptoms	Cubital tunnel pain, chronic numbness, and tingling in ulnar nerve distribution of the hand, tight wrist flexors, muscle weakness, feeling of hand falling asleep, weak grip
Treatment plan	Ice, stretch, anti-inflammatory medications, activity modification, bracing, surgery may be necessary and involves ulnar nerve transfer to relocate the ulnar nerve outside of cubital tunnel
Prevention strategies	Proper throwing mechanics, limit number of pitches per training session

Elbow Dislocation

An elbow dislocation is a serious medical emergency because the dislocation of the joint may also fracture the coronoid process or olecranon process. Often this injury happens when a person falls onto an outstretched hand or hyperextends the elbow. Athletes in sports such as wrestling and rodeo have a higher risk of elbow dislocation. In the case of any dislocation, it is especially important to splint the elbow as it lies and activate emergency medical services (EMS). The injury will often result in shock and can cause nerve or circulatory impairment. The elbow must be reduced by a medical professional. Elbow dislocations are discussed further in Table 8.6.

Table 8.6 Elbow dislocation

Mechanism of injury	Falling on an outstretched hand, hyperextension
Signs and symptoms	Deformity, pain, unable to move the elbow, decreased circulation, numbness or tingling in the hand or forearm
Treatment plan	Immobilize, check the pulse at the wrist, treat for shock, refer to emergency room (ER)
Prevention strategies	N/A

UCL Sprain

The UCL is most commonly sprained via traumatic or repetitive valgus force. This injury can also present as a chronic overuse injury due to poor throwing mechanics. Wrestling, baseball, and football are common activities that can result in this type of injury. The anterior band of the ligament is most commonly injured and can result in a great deal of disability. The UCL will often need time to heal, and conservative treatment is preferred over surgical intervention. This injury can be classified based on severity, ranging from first to third degree. If a third degree injury occurs, the surgical procedure used to reconstruct the UCL is known as Tommy John surgery. This procedure has been made famous due to the success of the surgery in baseball pitchers. Management of this condition is described in Table 8.7.

Table 8.7 UCL sprain

Signs and symptoms	Hearing or feeling a "pop," point tender over UCL, decreased range of motion, swelling over UCL
Treatment plan	Ice, rest, referral for second or third degree sprains, bracing, possibly surgery
Prevention strategies	Proper coaching for correct throwing mechanics

Bibliography

"AAOS—OrthoInfo." n.d. www.orthoinfo.aaos.org/ (accessed January 7, 2016).

"Diseases and Conditions." n.d. www.mayoclinic.org/diseases-conditions (accessed January 7, 2016).

Park, J.Y. 2015. *Sports Injuries to the Shoulder and Elbow.* Berlin, Germany: Springer.

CHAPTER 9

Wrist and Hand Injuries

Injuries to the wrist, hand, and fingers can result from everyday activities, work-related activities, participation in sports, or even fist fights. Injuries are commonly acute in nature but can also occur as a result of repetitive motion. The anatomy of the wrist and hand is quite complex and involves numerous joints and small structures. Knowledge of the anatomical structures is essential to understanding the complexities of the potential conditions that can occur in the wrist and hand. This chapter briefly reviews anatomy of the hand and wrist as well as common injuries and treatments.

Anatomy Review

Bone structure (see Figure 9.1):

Ulna

Radius

Trapezium (base of the first metacarpal)

Trapezoid (base of second metacarpal)

Capitate (base of the third metacarpal)

Hamate (base of fourth and fifth metacarpals)

Scaphoid or navicular (between radius and trapezium)

Lunate (between radius and capitate)

Triquetrum (distal to ulna)

Pisiform (palmer surface on triquetrum)

Metacarpals

Phalanges

Joints:

Distal radioulnar joint

Radiocarpal joint

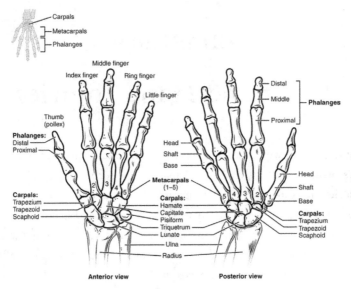

Figure 9.1 Bone anatomy of the hand

Intercarpal joints
Pisotriquetral joint
Carpometacarpal joints
Metacarpal phalangeal (MP) joints
Interphalangeal joint

Ligaments:
Ulnar collateral ligament (UCL; wrist and fingers)
Radial collateral ligament (wrist and fingers)
Transverse carpal ligament

Musculotendon structure (See Figure 9.2):
Flexor carpi ulnaris
Flexor carpi radialis
Palmaris longus
Extensor carpi radialis longus and brevis
Extensor carpi ulnaris
Extensor digitorum
Extensor indicis

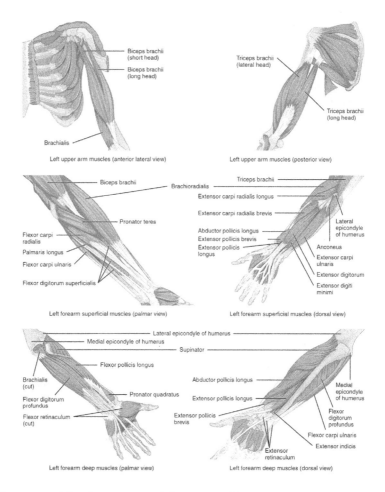

Figure 9.2 Muscle anatomy of the arm and hand

Palmar and dorsal interossei

Pronator quadratus

Other structure:

Anatomical Snuff Box

Borders:

Extensor pollicis longus

Abductor pollicis longus

Extensor pollicis brevis

Scaphoid (floor)

Contains:

Radial artery

Carpal Tunnel (see Figure 9.3)

Borders:

Proximal carpal bones (floor)

Transverse carpal ligament (roof)

Contains:

Flexor pollicis longus

Flexor digitorum superficialis

Flexor digitorum profundus

Flexor carpi radialis

Median nerve

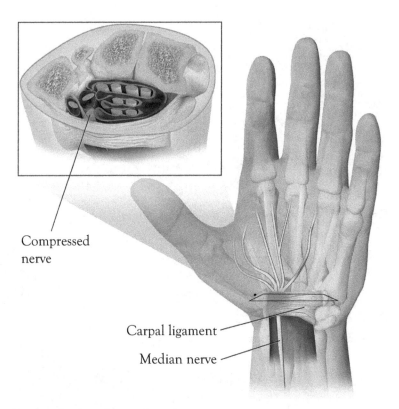

Compressed
nerve

Carpal ligament

Median nerve

Figure 9.3 Carpal tunnel syndrome

Tunnel of Guyon

Borders:

    Hook of hamate

    Pisiform

    Flexor retinaculum

    Pisohamate ligament

Contains:

    Ulnar nerve and artery

Thenar Eminence

Contains:

    Flexor pollicis brevis

    Adductor pollicis brevis

    Opponens pollicis

Hypothenar Eminenceeminence

Contains:

    Flexor digiti minimi

    Abductor digiti minimi

    Oppenens digiti minimi

Injuries

Metacarpal Fracture

The metacarpals are the long bones of the hands. There are several potential locations for fracture in the metacarpals; two of the most common are Bennett's fracture and Boxer's fracture. Bennett's fracture involves the first metacarpal base and the Boxer's fracture involves the fifth (and sometimes fourth) metacarpal. Most fractures to the metacarpals occur as a result of excessive force: by axial load, compression, or as a result of being stepped on. Minor fractures occur without displacement; however, if the trauma is due to angulation or rotational force, surgery may be necessary to reduce or fixate the bone. Additional considerations for this injury are described in Table 9.1.

Table 9.1 Metacarpal fracture

Mechanism of injury	Crushing, twisting, stepped on, or dropping something on your hand; a fall; direct contact in sport
Signs and symptoms	Limited hand function, pain, swelling, deformity over any metacarpal, finger may appear shorter, knuckle may look sunken
Treatment plan	X-ray, splint, possible surgery
Prevention strategies	N/A

Thumb UCL Sprain

The stability of the thumb is very important for grasping motions. The UCL is one of the most important ligaments in maintaining the stability of the thumb. A sprain of the UCL of the thumb can also be referred to as "skier's thumb" or "gamekeeper's thumb" (as this injury is commonly due to these activities). When a UCL sprain occurs, the tear can be partial or complete. In complicated cases, opposition of the thumb and other fingers may be lost. The UCL sprain can be debilitating and affect activities of daily living such as dressing, writing, and eating. Additional considerations are listed in Table 9.2.

Table 9.2 Thumb UCL sprain

Mechanism of injury	Falling on an outstretched hand forcing the thumb away from the hand, catching the thumb on a jersey, falling while skiing with a pole strapped to the hand
Signs and symptoms	Local pain, pain at the thumb joint, thumb feels weak when grasping, swelling
Treatment plan	Referral for second or third degree, splint or surgery may be needed
Prevention strategies	N/A

Mallet Finger

Mallet finger results from a rupture of the extensor tendon at the distal interphalangeal joint (DIP) of the tip of the finger. This injury often occurs in athletes who play sports such as football, basketball, and baseball, and is usually caused by a ball hitting the tip of the finger, commonly the index or middle finger(s). This injury can be further complicated if a chip of bone is pulled away with the tendon. Mallet finger is a difficult condition to treat due to failure of the patient to adhere to the prolonged splinting protocol. More information regarding this condition can be found in Table 9.3.

Table 9.3 Mallet finger

Signs and symptoms	Deformity, distal phalanx cannot be extended, swelling, pain, bruising
Treatment plan	Splint to maintain neutral position that *must* be worn at all times 6–8 weeks; rule out fracture with x-ray
Prevention strategies	N/A

Boutonniere Deformity

Boutonniere deformity is caused by a rupture of the extensor tendon at the proximal interphalangeal (PIP) joint, generally due to a blow to the tip of the finger. The injury is caused by forced flexion of the PIP joint or by being cut on the top of the finger. Chronically, the deformity can occur with arthritis. The primary indicator of a Boutonniere deformity is the inability to move the affected finger into extension. Treatment of this condition is provided in Table 9.4.

Table 9.4 Boutonniere deformity

Signs and symptoms	Deformity, cannot extend the finger at the PIP joint, the DIP joint will be extended, swelling, bruising, pain
Treatment plan	Splinting, refer to a medical doctor quickly because the tendons will tighten as time goes on, possible surgery to fix extensor tendon
Prevention strategies	N/A

Swan Neck Deformity

A Swan neck deformity occurs when there is a rupture of the volar plate under the PIP joint. The resulting deformity leaves the PIP joint sunken, and the DIP joint is forced into flexion. This deformity literally looks like the head and neck of a swan. Treatment involves referral and potential surgery and is further described in Table 9.5.

Table 9.5 Swan neck deformity

Mechanism of injury	Blow to tip of finger, hyperextension, inflammatory disease: commonly rheumatoid arthritis, laxity of the volar plate
Signs and symptoms	Deformity, middle joint of the finger is sunken in, DIP is stuck in flexion
Treatment plan	Referral, treating underlying disorder, splinting

MP, DIP, and PIP Sprains

Sprains to the joints of the fingers, also called "jammed fingers," occur frequently as a result of participation in sports. A sprain to the MP joint, DIP joint, or PIP joint, can be difficult to distinguish from a fracture. When an athlete sprains any of these structures, an x-ray is necessary to rule out an avulsion fracture. Signs and symptoms, as well as management strategies are described in Table 9.6.

Table 9.6 MP, DIP, and PIP sprains

Mechanism of injury	Direct blow, axial load, catching a finger on clothing, falling
Signs and symptoms	Pain at joint, swelling, bruising, decreased strength, decreased range of motion, decreased function of the finger
Treatment plan	Splint, ice, encourage range-of-motion activities if fracture is not suspected
Prevention strategies	N/A

MP, DIP, and PIP Dislocation

Dislocation of the MP, DIP, and PIP joints involves the same mechanism as a sprain but the joint is displaced. There is generally a potential for a fracture in addition to the joint displacement; so generally some type of imaging will have to be performed in order to determine if a fracture has occurred. As with any dislocation, reduction should only be performed by a qualified medical professional. In rare cases, surgery may be required. Table 9.7 describes these dislocations in further detail.

Table 9.7 MP, DIP, and PIP dislocation

Mechanism of injury	Direct blow, axial load, catching a finger on clothing, falling
Signs and symptoms	Deformity, inability to move the joint, swelling, pain, bruising
Treatment plan	Ice, splint, reduction, x-ray
Prevention strategies	N/A

Phalanx Fracture

The fingers are made up of multiple smaller bones called phalanx. The thumb has two phalanx, while the index through the pinky fingers have three. A fracture to a phalanx is generally caused by a direct blow to the finger and commonly co-occurs with a sprained or dislocated finger. In the affected finger, the patient will feel pain, have decreased function, and often there will be a noticeable bone deformity. Treatment protocols vary depending on the injury and are described in Table 9.8.

Table 9.8 Phalanx fracture

Mechanism of injury	Hit on the tip of finger, dislocation, direct blow
Signs and symptoms	Pain, deformity, swelling, decreased function
Treatment plan	Splint, ice, no treatment, possible surgery
Prevention strategies	N/A

Subungual Hematoma

A subungual hematoma is more commonly referred to as simply "blood underneath the fingernail." This results from a direct blow to the fingertip or smashing the distal phalanx with an object such as a hammer. The person will have severe pain and pressure under the nail. Typically, the nail will eventually fall off as it grows out but this may take several months. Table 9.9 provides further details on subungual hematomas.

Trigger Finger

Tendons are cord-like structures that normally glide smoothly through a sheath that surrounds them. Trigger finger involves a deformity that results

Table 9.9 Subungual hematoma

Signs and symptoms	Blood under the fingernail, throbbing pain, and pressure under nail
Treatment plan	Drill the nail to relieve the pressure and blood, apply ice, most likely to lose the nail as it grows out
Prevention strategies	N/A

from the irritation and thickening of the flexor tendon sheath. When the sheath thickens, the tendon "sticks" as the patient attempts to flex the finger. As the patient flexes the finger, the tendon sticks, and the finger releases, often with a snap. The condition worsens, over time and the finger will not let go, so movement into extension must be done manually. Trigger finger is more common in women and in patients who also have diabetes. It most commonly affects the thumb, ring finger, or middle finger. This condition may be painful and often conservative treatment fails. Table 9.10 describes mechanisms, signs and symptoms, and treatment options.

Table 9.10 Trigger finger

Mechanism of injury	Overuse due to repetitive gripping motion, inflammatory diseases, diabetes
Signs and symptoms	Progresses from mild to severe; stiffness, inability to move finger into flexion, pain, palpation of a node (bump) under the affected finger, symptoms worse in the morning
Treatment plan	Anti-inflammatory medications , splint, stretching, steroid injection, possible surgery
Prevention strategies	N/A

De Quervain's Syndrome

De Quervain's syndrome is tenosynovitis of the abductor pollicis longus and the extensor pollicis brevis tendons of the thumb. The most common mechanism is overuse and commonly seen in those who play racket sports, garden, or golf. Repetitive motions associated with these activities can cause the sheath around the tendons of the thumb to become irritated and thickened, causing pain when used. De Quervain's syndrome also seems to be more common in middle-aged women. This condition may be diagnosed by isolating the involved muscles and crepitus can be felt or heard at the joint. Further details are mentioned in Table 9.11.

Table 9.11 De Quervain's syndrome

Mechanism of injury	Repetitive hand or wrist movements, direct blow to the tendons, inflammatory diseases
Signs and symptoms	Pain on the tendons on the top of the thumb, pain with movement of wrist, pain with use of thumb, pain with making a fist or grasping items, swelling, a sticking sensation when you move the thumb
Treatment plan	Ice, anti-inflammatory medications, rest, possible splint, followed by strengthening exercises
Prevention strategies	N/A

Carpal Tunnel Syndrome

Carpal tunnel syndrome results from the median nerve being pinched or compressed as it passes through the wrist to the hand. Generally, people who are at risk for this condition include individuals who use their hands daily for fine motor skills, such as factory employees, cosmetologists, and office workers. This condition is often confused with tendonitis. The difference between the two is that carpal tunnel syndrome will result in numbness and weakness in the median nerve distribution of the hand. Consultation with a medical professional can help determine the most appropriate course of treatment. Additional information is mentioned in Table 9.12.

Table 9.12 Carpal tunnel syndrome

Mechanism of injury	Repetitive motions, sleeping with wrists in a flexed position, improper ergonomics at workstation, anatomical abnormalities, underlying health problems, pregnancy
Signs and symptoms	Pain, hand numbness and tingling, weakness following median nerve pathway in the hand (thumb, index, and middle fingers)
Treatment plan	Rest, brace, anti-inflammatory medications, night splint, surgery may be needed
Prevention strategies	Proper ergonomics at work, taking breaks, wrist stretches, improved posture

Wrist Ganglion Cyst

Ganglion cysts are fluid filled sacs that occur under the skin, commonly on the top of the wrist and occur when the sheath around tendon becomes inflamed and fills with fluid. Cysts can range from the size of a pea to nearly an inch in diameter. Large cysts may interfere with wrist motions. Often there is no mechanism of injury but overuse may be a contributing cause (playing racquet sports or golf). There are a number of treatments that can be effective in reducing the ganglion, but often the cyst will disappear and reappear on its own. Recurrent cysts may require surgical intervention. Further information regarding this condition can be found in Table 9.13.

Table 9.13 Wrist ganglion cyst

Signs and symptoms	Notable bump on back of hand or wrist, may be symptom free, rarely painful, decreased range of motion if larger, discomfort doing push-ups, may mimic a wrist sprain
Treatment plan	Usually goes away on its own, corticosteroid injection, possible surgery for removal
Prevention strategies	N/A

Scaphoid Fracture

The scaphoid bone is located within the anatomical snuffbox of the wrist at the base of the thumb. Fracture to the scaphoid can be the result of acute injury, such as a fall, or due to chronic repetitive motions that place excessive stress on the bone (e.g., heavy bench press). Unfortunately, a scaphoid fracture often will not present on an initial x-ray, and rate of healing is very slow. Complications of a scaphoid fracture are common, usually due to a nonunion or avascular necrosis (disruption of the blood supply to the bone resulting in tissue death). If the bone does not heal with immobilization, surgical intervention may be required. Additional information may be found in Table 9.14.

Table 9.14 Scaphoid fracture

Mechanism of injury	Falling on an outstretched hand, wrist hyperextension, weight lifting, motor vehicle accidents
Signs and symptoms	Apparent wrist sprain that does not improve, pain in anatomical snuff box at the base of the thumb, pain with thumb or wrist movements
Treatment plan	Immobilization, ice, may need cast (above elbow to stop supination or pronation), surgery
Prevention strategies	Use of a wrist brace during risky activity (snowboarding, skiing, rollerblading, etc.)

Triangular Fibrocartilage Complex Tear

The triangular fibrocartilage complex (TFCC) is a fibrous cartilage disc that lies between the bones of the forearm and the wrist and on the pinky side. The purpose of this structure is to provide stability during grasping activities. Tears of the TFCC can either be acute or due to chronic overuse of the wrist and hand. Injury or inflammation of the TFCC varies in severity but can be rather debilitating. An acute tear or sprain to this cartilaginous complex is often the result of falling on an outstretched hand where the cartilage is forcefully pinched between the ulna, lunate, and capitate. The patient will notice significant pain at the ulnar–carpal space. Conservative treatment is usually recommended and is explained in Table 9.15.

Table 9.15 TFCC tear

Mechanism of injury	Acute—falling on an outstretched hand, forces over rotation of the hand or wrist Chronic—degenerative overtime
Signs and symptoms	Chronic wrist pain, pain at ulna or carpal space, pain with wrist motions, clicking in the wrist, swelling, loss of grip strength
Treatment plan	Referral, splint or cast to allow for structures to heal, anti-inflammatory medications, injections, possible surgery
Prevention strategies	Use of a wrist brace during risky activity (snowboarding, skiing, rollerblading, etc.)

Carpal or Wrist Sprain

The wrist is made of numerous tiny bones that are connected by a plethora of ligaments and other soft tissues. Any activity that results in overstretching of these ligaments can result in a sprain. Sprains can range in severity from first to third degree depending on the force applied to the wrist. If the injury is severe, it can limit activity equally as much as a fracture. The injury may require an x-ray to rule out a fracture. Treatment protocol, as listed in Table 9.16, is determined based on imaging outcomes and specific functional tests performed by a medical professional.

Table 9.16 Carpal or wrist sprain

Mechanism of injury	Wrist hyperextension or hyperflexion, falling on an out-stretched hand
Signs and symptoms	Pain with wrist movement, general weakness, unable to perform daily activities, swelling, point tenderness over injured ligaments
Treatment plan	Rest, ice, splint, anti-inflammatory medications, referral to rule out a fracture, followed by strengthening exercises
Prevention strategies	Use of a wrist brace during risky activities (snowboarding, skiing, rollerblading, etc.)

Colles Fracture

The most commonly fractured bone of the arm is the radius. When a fracture occurs at the distal end, closer to the wrist, it is considered a Colles fracture. The fracture typically occurs about one inch from the end of the bone and is denoted by a dorsal displacement of the involved hand. The mechanism generally involves falling on an outstretched arm and is characterized by immediate deformity. The fracture can be further classified, based on severity, which will determine the treatment plan. This condition is considered a medical emergency due to potential for circulatory compromise, and the patient should be taken to an emergency room as soon as possible. Further information regarding this injury can be found in Table 9.17.

Table 9.17 Colles fracture

Mechanism of injury	Falling in an extended wrist
Signs and symptoms	Immediate severe pain, deformity, pain with finger movement, swelling
Treatment plan	Splint, check pulse, emergency room referral, cast, possible surgery
Prevention strategies	Use of a wrist brace during risky activities (snowboarding, skiing, rollerblading, etc.)

Smith's Fracture

The Smith's fracture, also known as the reverse Colles fracture, is a radial fracture that presents with a volar displacement of the injured hand. Smith's fractures are less common than Colles fractures because of the rare nature of the mechanism of injury: falling with the wrist flexed. Deformity will be immediately apparent as with the Colles fracture. This condition is also considered a medical emergency due to potential circulatory impairment. It is essential to recognize this condition and refer as soon as possible. Table 9.18 further explains the signs, symptoms, and treatment for this condition.

Table 9.18 Smith's fracture

Mechanism of injury	Falling on a flexed wrist
Signs and symptoms	Immediate severe pain, swelling, deformity, pain with finger movement
Treatment plan	Splint, check pulse, emergency room referral, cast, possible surgery
Prevention strategies	Use of a wrist brace during risky activities (snowboarding, skiing, rollerblading, etc.)

Bibliography

"AAOS—OrthoInfo." n.d. www.orthoinfo.aaos.org/ (accessed January 7, 2016).

Anderson, M.K. 2011. *Fundamentals of Sports Injury Management*. Philadelphia, PA: Lippincott Williams & Wilkins.

"Diseases and Conditions." n.d. www.mayoclinic.org/diseases-conditions (accessed January 7, 2016).

Isaacs, J.E., and M.D. Miller. 2015. *Sports Hand and Wrist Injuries*. Philadelphia, PA: Elsevier.

CHAPTER 10

Cervical Spine Injuries

Cervical spine injuries can range from minor conditions to catastrophic or life-threatening circumstances. The cervical spine is among the most important structures in the body as it includes and protects organs and structures vital to sustaining life. It is essential to understand the complexity of the anatomy of this region and appreciate the importance of small bony structures and surrounding musculature. This chapter describes the anatomical regions of the cervical spine and identifies common complications involving these areas.

Anatomy Review

Bone structure (see Figure 10.1):

C1

> Atlas

C2

> Axis, odontoid process or dens
> Transverse foramen

C3, C4, C5

> Bifurcated spinous process

C6–C7

Ligaments (see Figure 10.2):

> Anterior longitudinal ligament (anterior to vertebral bodies)
> Posterior longitudinal ligament (posterior to vertebral bodies)
> Ligamentum flavum
> Intertransverse ligament
> Interspinous ligament
> Supraspinous ligament

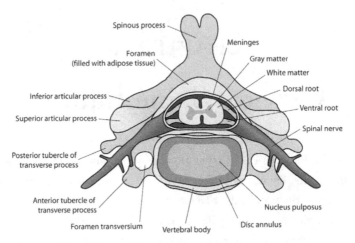

Figure 10.1 Cervical vertebrae anatomy

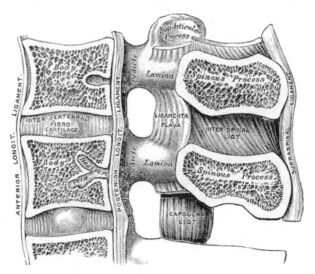

Figure 10.2 Ligament anatomy of the spine

Musculotendon structure (see Figure 10.3):

Scalenes

Anterior, middle, posterior

Sternocleidomastoid

Trapezius

Longissimus

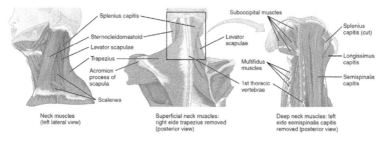

Figure 10.3 Muscle anatomy of the neck

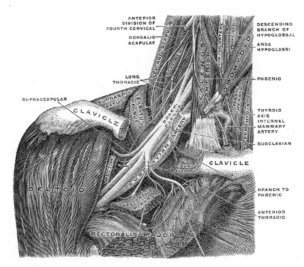

Figure 10.4 Brachial plexus

Iliocostalis

Spinalis

Other structure:

Intervertebral discs

Brachial plexus (see Figure 10.4)

Injuries

Torticollis

Torticollis is an abnormal tilt or rotation to the neck and head. It is also known as "wry neck" and can be named according to the direction of rotation of the neck. Torticollis typically presents with muscle spasms resulting in the neck being stiff and "stuck" in a slightly rotated position. Most commonly, the sternocleidomastoid and trapezius muscles are involved. Many conditions can lead to torticollis, and the underlying cause must be determined. Additional information can be found in Table 10.1.

Table 10.1 Torticollis

Mechanism of injury	Sleeping on improper pillows, muscle spasm, congenital disorders, certain medical conditions
Signs and symptoms	Neck stiffness, neck or head in tilted or rotated position, muscle pain
Treatment plan	Determining cause, stretching, heat treatment, massage
Prevention Strategies	N/A

Muscle Strain and Sprains

Many soft tissues surround the cervical spine to allow this region of the body a large range of motion; thus, with a large amount of mobility comes increased risk of injury. Muscle strains can occur acutely, commonly with whiplash, or they can occur due to chronic repetitive activities. Typically, muscle strains and ligament sprains occur at the same time and are commonly treated the same way. Additional information about neck strains can be found in Table 10.2.

Table 10.2 Muscle strain and sprains

Mechanism of injury	Poor posture, motor vehicle accident or whiplash, poor sleeping position, straining while carrying a heavy object, lifting weights, falling from a height
Signs and symptoms	Pain with neck movement, stiff neck, headache, muscles soreness in the upper back or arms, difficulty sleeping
Treatment plan	Ice, heat, stretching, anti-inflammatory medications, followed by strengthening and postural improvements
Prevention strategies	Improve posture, neck stretching and strengthening

Vertebral Fracture

Seven vertebrae make up the cervical portion of the spinal column. These vertebrae serve to support the head and protect the spinal cord. Fractures of the vertebrae typically result from high-velocity impact commonly seen in falls, contact sports, or motor vehicle accidents. Injury to the cervical vertebra can lead to subsequent damage to the spinal cord, causing permanent loss of function of the lower extremities (paralysis). All neck injuries need to be treated as medical emergencies until further evaluation can be conducted by a medical professional. See Table 10.3 for more details concerning cervical fractures.

Table 10.3 Vertebra fracture

Mechanism of injury	Axial loading, axial load with rotation, hyperextension
Signs and symptoms	Cervical pain, extremity pain, numbness in extremities, decreased strength in extremities, loss of bladder or bowel control, decreased movement in neck, muscle spasm
Treatment plan	Immediate spinal immobilization, spine boarding, x-ray, other treatments will depend on which vertebra is fractured and what other damage is involved, cervical bracing, surgery
Prevention strategies	Wearing appropriate sports equipment, using proper tackling techniques, wearing seat belts, avoiding diving into shallow water

Spinal Cord Damage

Injury to the spinal cord is very serious and, often, below the lesion level, there is permanent reduction of sensory and motor function. The spinal cord can be injured in numerous ways, including partial or complete lacerations, bruises, and compression by other surrounding structures. A laceration to the spinal cord occurs when the cord is cut, usually as a result of a fracture or dislocation and the involved vertebral bone ends pierce cord either partially or completely and often results in permanent damage. The spinal cord is also susceptible to contusions, or bruising, from any force that displaces the vertebrae and can result in temporary or permanent paralysis. A less severe form of spinal cord injury, "spinal cord shock," results from a mild contusion to cord that initially presents as paralysis but is transient and without permanent damage. Regardless of perceived severity, any person who has fallen; been in a motor vehicle accident; or has receives a hard blow to the head, neck, or back and complains of neck pain with symptoms of numbness or tingling in the extremities needs to be treated with the utmost precautions. Emergency medical services (EMS) needs to be activated immediately. Do not move the victim without knowing how to perform proper spinal immobilization and spine boarding techniques. Victim should be immobilized until evaluated by a medical professional. See Table 10.4 for details concerning spinal cord injuries.

Table 10.4 *Spinal cord damage*

Mechanism of injury	Axial load, displaced vertebral fracture, motor vehicle accident, falls, blow to the spine, severe whiplash, disc injury, acts of violence
Signs and symptoms	Inability to move limbs, numb limbs, initial severe back pain, loss of bladder or bowel functions, signs and symptoms vary depending on the level of the cervical cord damage
Treatment plan	Activating EMS, spinal immobilization, spine boarding, x-ray, surgery
Prevention strategies	Wearing appropriate sports equipment, using proper tackling techniques, wearing seat belts, avoiding diving into shallow water

Burners or Stingers

A burner or stinger is the result of an overstretch or compression of the nerves in the brachial plexus of the neck. This injury is a common occurrence in athletes who tackle, especially football defensive players and linebackers. Generally, a stinger occurs when there is traction or compression of the brachial plexus as a result of the neck being forced sideways or by a direct blow to Erb's point, which lies halfway between the neck and shoulder. This injury often results in numbness, weakness,

Table 10.5 *Burners or stingers*

Signs and symptoms	Burning or tingling sensation around the neck, down the arm, or into the hand; numbness or tingling surrounding the arm, but only affects one arm; this does not follow dermatomal pattern, and may cause muscle weakness or point tenderness over Erb's point
Treatment plan	Numbness or tingling usually resolves in 1–2 minutes without intervention; decreased strength and range of motion may linger; more severe injury may result in permanent nerve damage
Prevention strategies	Neck roll padding or cowboy collar for football or sports involving shoulder pads

and tingling in the shoulder, which usually resolve within a few minutes. The greater the number of times this injury occurs, the longer the symptoms will last. It is essential to cease participation in activity while symptoms are present, as the athlete will not be able to adequately protect a numb or weak shoulder from further injury. Table 10.5 gives further guidance for treating this condition.

Cervical Disc Pathology

Due to the large range of motion and mobility of the neck, the cervical discs are susceptible to sustaining repeated stress and, over time, degeneration may present as neck pain with radicular symptoms down into the shoulder, arm, and hand. Injury to the discs of the neck are commonly referred to bulging, herniated, or slipped. As we age, disc pathology becomes more likely because the discs lose some of their water content and overall integrity. The majority of cervical disc injuries occur in C5–C6. A herniated disc can range in severity from mild to severe, depending on the degree of disc displacement. Pathology begins with the nucleus of the disc pushing out on the outer rings of the annulus and progresses to where the disc pushes onto peripheral nerves and beyond. Additional description and the treatment of this condition can be found in Table 10.6.

Table 10.6 Cervical disc pathology

Mechanism of injury	Neck flexion with rotation, repetitive movement, improper lifting techniques, axial load
Signs and symptoms	General neck pain, pain radiating down the arm to the hand, decreased sensation in specific areas of the upper extremities, decreased reflexes in area, signs and symptoms reproduced with neck flexion or neck compression, weak arm or hand muscles
Treatment plan	Rest, ice, anti-inflammatory medications, extension exercises
Prevention strategies	N/A

Spinal Stenosis

Spinal stenosis is the narrowing of the spinal canal, which causes impingement and places pressure on the spinal cord. Spinal stenosis typically

Table 10.7 Spinal stenosis

Mechanism of injury	Congenital or any change in vertebrae, osteophytes, bone spurs, disc pathology, tumors, hemorrhage
Signs and symptoms	Possibly symptom free or pain down the arm, sensory changes like burning and tingling into the arm and hand, motor changes such as decreased strength, muscle atrophy
Treatment plan	Anti-inflammatory medications, muscle relaxants, and other prescription medications; steroid injections; in severe cases possible surgery to make more room for the spinal cord
Prevention strategies	N/A

occurs either in the neck or the lumbar region of the spinal column. The narrowing can be caused by several factors, including repetitive activities that lead to osteoarthritis and eventually changes in the structure of the bones. Spinal stenosis typically occurs in people over the age of 50 years. Additional information about spinal stenosis can be found in Table 10.7.

Bibliography

"AAOS—OrthoInfo." n.d. www.orthoinfo.aaos.org/ (accessed January 7, 2016).

"Diseases and Conditions." n.d. www.mayoclinic.org/diseases-conditions (accessed January 7, 2016).

Gorse, K.M. 2010. *Emergency Care in Athletic Training.* Philadelphia, PA: F.A. Davis.

Hopkins, G. 2015. *Sports Injuries: Prevention, Management and Risk Factors.* New York: Nova Publishers.

Micheli, L.J., C.J. Stein, M. O'Brien, and P. D'Hemecourt. 2014. *Spinal Injuries and Conditions in Young Athletes.* New York: Springer.

CHAPTER 11

Head Injuries

Head injuries are common in sports and should be treated as serious injuries. The majority of head injuries occur by direct blunt force, including hitting the head on an object, blunt-force trauma, motor vehicle accidents, falls, or collision with another person. The brain is a soft structure that sits within a hard bony cranium. The skull provides protection and support for the brain but often the mechanical forces that result from a fall or direct blow are greater than the durability of the skull. Furthermore, any direct force to the skull will be transmitted to the brain, which consequently bounces around inside the hard skull. Thus, any injury to the bony anatomy of the skull also creates potential for a brain injury. This chapter provides a brief review of cranial anatomy and outlines specific structures that are susceptible to injury.

Anatomy Review

Bone structure (see Figure 11.1):

Frontal

Parietal

Sphenoid

Temporal

Occipital

Nasal

Maxilla

Mandible

Zygomatic arch

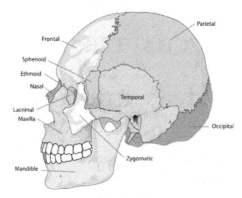

Figure 11.1 Bone anatomy of the skull

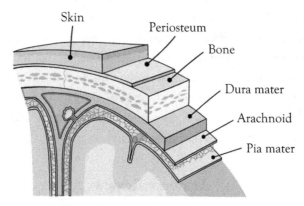

Figure 11.2 Meninges

Other structures (see Figure 11.2):
    Dura mater—lines the skull
    Arachnoid mater—middle lining
    Cerebrospinal fluid
    Pia mater—lines the brain

Injuries

Skull Fracture

Any large force to the head can result in a skull fracture. Depending on the amount and direction of the force to the head, there are many types of cranial fractures that may result. Fractures can be classified as closed or open, where open fractures break through the surface of the skin. Skull fractures commonly result in either a depression fracture or basilar skull fracture. Depression fractures are notable due to a depressed or sunken appearance, wherein the fracture moves inward toward the brain. Basilar skull fractures involve the base of the skull and commonly present with blood pooling behind the ears and under the eyes. Skull fractures should be treated as medical emergencies and evaluated immediately by a medical professional. Additional information, including signs and symptoms, can be found in Table 11.1.

Table 11.1 Skull fracture

Mechanism of injury	Direct blow to the head, falling, motor vehicle accident, sports trauma
Signs and symptoms	Pain at the site of impact, bleeding from the wound, bruising that pools under the eyes (raccoon eyes), bruising behind the ears (battle sign), noted depression in the skull, cerebrospinal fluid coming out of the nose or ears, headache, tinnitus, nausea, irritability, confusion, disorientation, dizziness, loss of consciousness, memory loss
Treatment plan	Mild fracture—pain medications Severe fracture—neurosurgery
Prevention strategies	Wearing protective equipment during risky activities, wearing seat belts

Closed Head Injury, Concussion, or Mild Traumatic Brain Injury

Closed head injuries, or concussions, usually occur as a result of a blow to the head. The brain is housed within the skull, and when the head is struck with force, it can cause the brain to bounce around within the hard structure of the skull. Concussions do not always result in a loss of consciousness. Signs and symptoms include immediate impairment of brain function, which can present in a multitude of ways (memory, coordination, emotional control, etc. See Table 11.2). Closed head injuries can lead to lifelong neurological, cognitive, and psychological impairment. The effects of concussions are cumulative in nature and the damage becomes

Table 11.2 Closed head injury, concussion, or mild traumatic brain injury

Mechanism of injury	Direct blow to the head, falling, motor vehicle accident, sports trauma, focal or diffused trauma
Signs and symptoms	Initial symptoms: headache, amnesia, ringing in the ears, nausea, irritability, confusion, disorientation, dizziness, blurred vision, seizures, loss of consciousness, coma Secondary symptoms: concentration difficulty, photophobia, sleep disturbance, depression, anxiety, changes to personality
Treatment plan	Rest the brain, *avoid* brain stimulus such as video games; screen time; *avoid* giving aspirin or other medications that could thin the blood unless directed by a medical professional; *avoid* drinking alcohol or caffeine, which thin the blood; *no* return to activity until all signs and symptoms are gone and the athlete is able to pass concussion protocol testing *Follow-up in the emergency room is needed in cases of*: increased headache, increased drowsiness, increased dizziness, increased confusion or disorientation, nausea or vomiting getting worse, vision changes, loss of memory, starting of convulsions, starting of slurred speech, increased ringing in the ears, face numbness, difficulty or inability to be aroused from sleep
Prevention strategies	Wearing protective equipment during risky activities, do not return to activity until cleared by a medical professional

increasingly severe. Furthermore, once an individual has sustained one concussion, he or she is more likely to sustain another. Information regarding management of this condition can be found in Table 11.2.

Epidural Hematoma

Epidural hematomas are a type of traumatic brain injury that present with blood pooling between the dura mater and the skull. Commonly, the bleed occurs on the side of brain where the impact took place. The pressure placed on the brain within the intracranial space causes the brain to shift; this occurs quickly because the source of the bleed is from an artery. Thus, signs and symptoms of epidural hematomas present very quickly after injury, usually within 10 minutes to a few hours. Epidural hematomas cause increased pressure within the intracranial space and the patient presents with quickly worsening symptoms. Early recognition and activation of emergency medical services (EMS) is a priority because the pressure on the brain must be alleviated as soon as possible. This can only be accomplished via prompt neurosurgery; but if successful the prognosis is good. Further information concerning epidural hematomas can be found in Table 11.3.

Table 11.3 Epidural hematoma

Mechanism of injury	Direct blow to the head, acceleration–deceleration injuries, coup force, motor vehicle accidents, sports trauma, assault
Signs and symptoms	Initial lucid interval followed by unequal or fixed pupils, increased heart rate, lucid intervals, poor eye tracking, irregular respirations, severe headache, projectile vomit
Treatment plan	Need surgical release of pressure, cognitive rehabilitation
Prevention strategies	Wearing protective equipment during risky activities, wearing seat belts

Subdural Hematoma

Subdural hematomas are a type of traumatic brain injury that present with blood pooling between the dura mater and the pia mater. Commonly, the bleed occurs on the opposite side of impact. Subdural hematomas result from a ruptured cranial vein; thus, the individual will present with signs and symptoms much more slowly than in the case of an epidural hematoma. Subdural hematomas can be classified as acute, subacute, or chronic depending on how quickly signs and symptoms develop, which may not become evident for several hours to days or weeks postinjury. As a result, the venous bleed can actually be deadlier than epidural hematoma arterial bleed because an individual may not relate symptoms to a head trauma that possibly occurred weeks before and delay seeking treatment. Further information regarding this condition is described in Table 11.4.

Chronic Traumatic Encephalopathy

Chronic traumatic encephalopathy (CTE) is a devastating condition that involves progressive neurological deterioration caused by repeated blows

Table 11.4 Subdural hematoma

Mechanism of injury	Direct blow to the head, acceleration–deceleration injuries, contrecoup force, motor vehicle accidents, sports trauma, assault
Signs and symptoms	Unconsciousness, then lucid intervals, headache, dizziness, nausea, unequal pupils, disorientation, sleepiness, decreased level of consciousness, decreased pulse, decreased respirations, convulsions, weakness, balance disturbance, personality change, visual changes, loss of appetite, altered breathing pattern
Treatment plan	Dependent on the size and rate of the bleed Small bleeds—monitor Large bleeds—neurosurgery
Prevention strategies	Wearing protective equipment during risky activities, wearing seat belts

to the head. The condition was originally deemed similar to "Dementia Pugilistica," which was found initially in boxers. The disease has primarily been found in post mortem American football and hockey players. Continuous repetitive trauma triggers progressive degeneration of the brain tissue, including the buildup of an abnormal protein called Tau. Tau proteins are thought to causes changes to the brain over time, but, unfortunately, the presence of the protein can only be detected upon autopsy. The development of symptoms due to these proteins may occur months, years, or even decades post-trauma(s). The majority of individuals who have been found to have suffered from CTE committed suicide and their families have donated their brains to science for further research. Signs and symptoms of this condition are discussed in Table 11.5.

Table 11.5 Chronic traumatic encephalopathy

Mechanism of injury	Continuous repetitive trauma from repeated blows to the head
Signs and symptoms	Memory loss, confusion, impaired judgment, impulse control problems, aggression, depression, and, eventually, progressive dementia
Treatment plan	There is no treatment currently for CTE
Prevention strategies	Research is being conducted to determine whether CTE can be prevented

Bibliography

"AAOS—OrthoInfo." n.d. www.orthoinfo.aaos.org/ (accessed January 7, 2016).

Cantu, R.C., and M. Hyman. 2012. *Concussions and Our Kids: America's Leading Expert on How to Protect Young Athletes and Keep Sports Safe.* Boston, MA: Houghton Mifflin Harcourt.

"Diseases and Conditions." n.d. www.mayoclinic.org/diseases-conditions (accessed January 7, 2016).

Kirk, M., M. Wiser, S. Fainaru, and M. Fainaura-Wada. 2013. *League of Denial: The NFL's Concussion Crisis.*

Petraglia, A.L., J.E. Bailes, and A.L. Day. 2015. *Handbook of Neurological Sports Medicine: Concussion and Other Nervous System Injuries in the Athlete.* Champaign, IL: Human Kinetics.

Index

THIS TITLE IS FROM OUR HEALTH, WELLNESS, AND EXERCISE SCIENCE COLLECTION

Abigail Larson, Southern Utah University, *Editor*

Fuel for Sport: The Basics
by Abigail Larson

*Strategies for Sport Nutrition Success: A Practical Guide to
Improving Performance Through Nutrition*
by Abigail Larson

Momentum Press is one of the leading book publishers in the field of engineering, mathematics, health, and applied sciences. Momentum Press offers over 30 collections, including Aerospace, Biomedical, Civil, Environmental, Nanomaterials, Geotechnical, and many others.

Momentum Press is actively seeking collection editors as well as authors. For more information about becoming an MP author or collection editor, please visit
http://www.momentumpress.net/contact

Announcing Digital Content Crafted by Librarians

Momentum Press offers digital content as authoritative treatments of advanced engineering topics by leaders in their field. Hosted on ebrary, MP provides practitioners, researchers, faculty, and students in engineering, science, and industry with innovative electronic content in sensors and controls engineering, advanced energy engineering, manufacturing, and materials science.

Momentum Press offers library-friendly terms:

- perpetual access for a one-time fee
- no subscriptions or access fees required
- unlimited concurrent usage permitted
- downloadable PDFs provided
- free MARC records included
- free trials

The **Momentum Press** digital library is very affordable, with no obligation to buy in future years.

For more information, please visit **www.momentumpress.net/library** or to set up a trial in the US, please contact **mpsales@globalepress.com.**

CPSIA information can be obtained
at www.ICGtesting.com
Printed in the USA
JSHW041100201220
10398JS00002B/37

9 781944 749392